CW00521457

Plant-Based Diet Cookbook with Pictures

Delicious, Whole-Food, Plant-Based Recipes to Cook Every Day for Busy People

Michael Gill

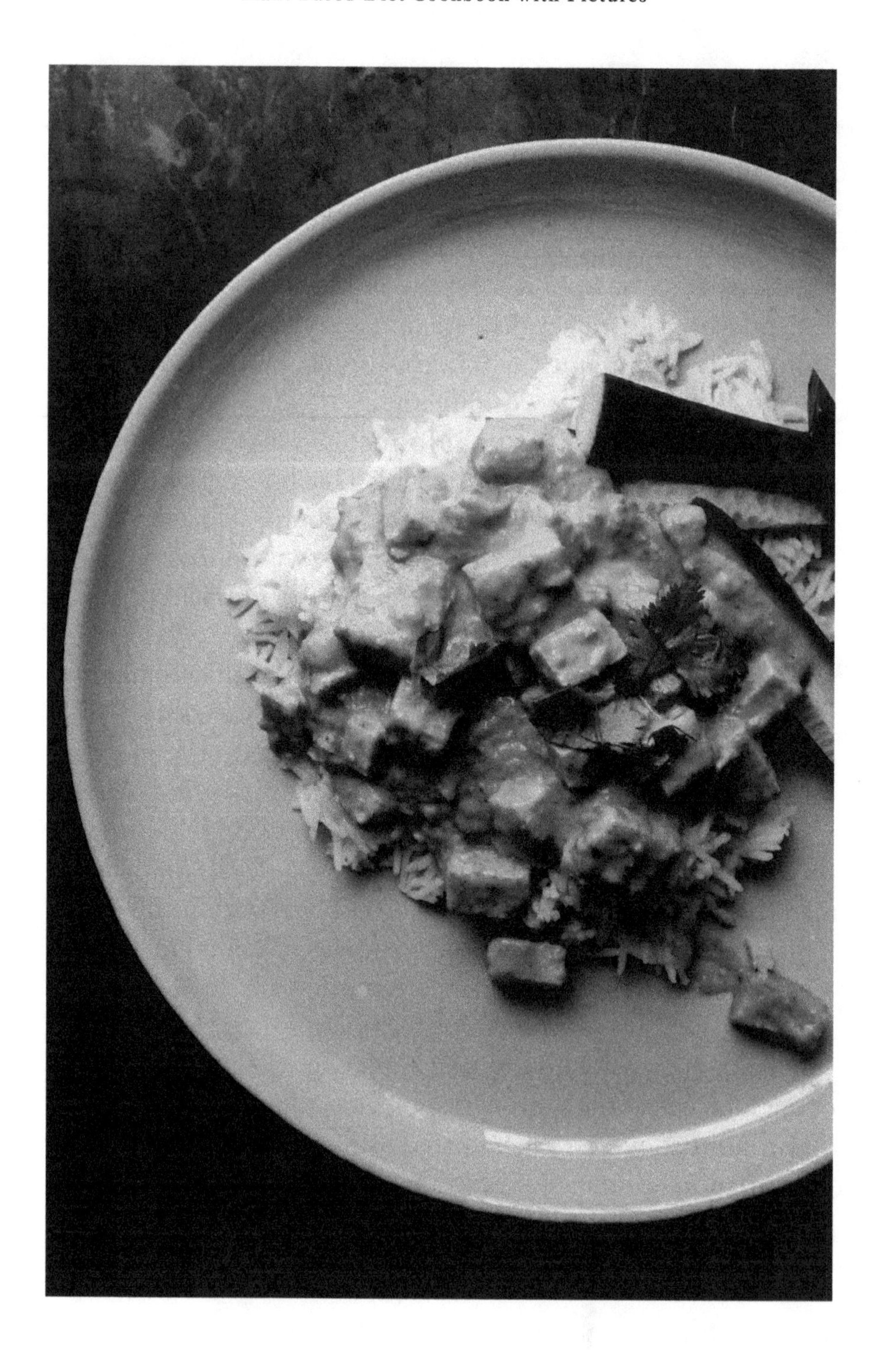

Table of Contents

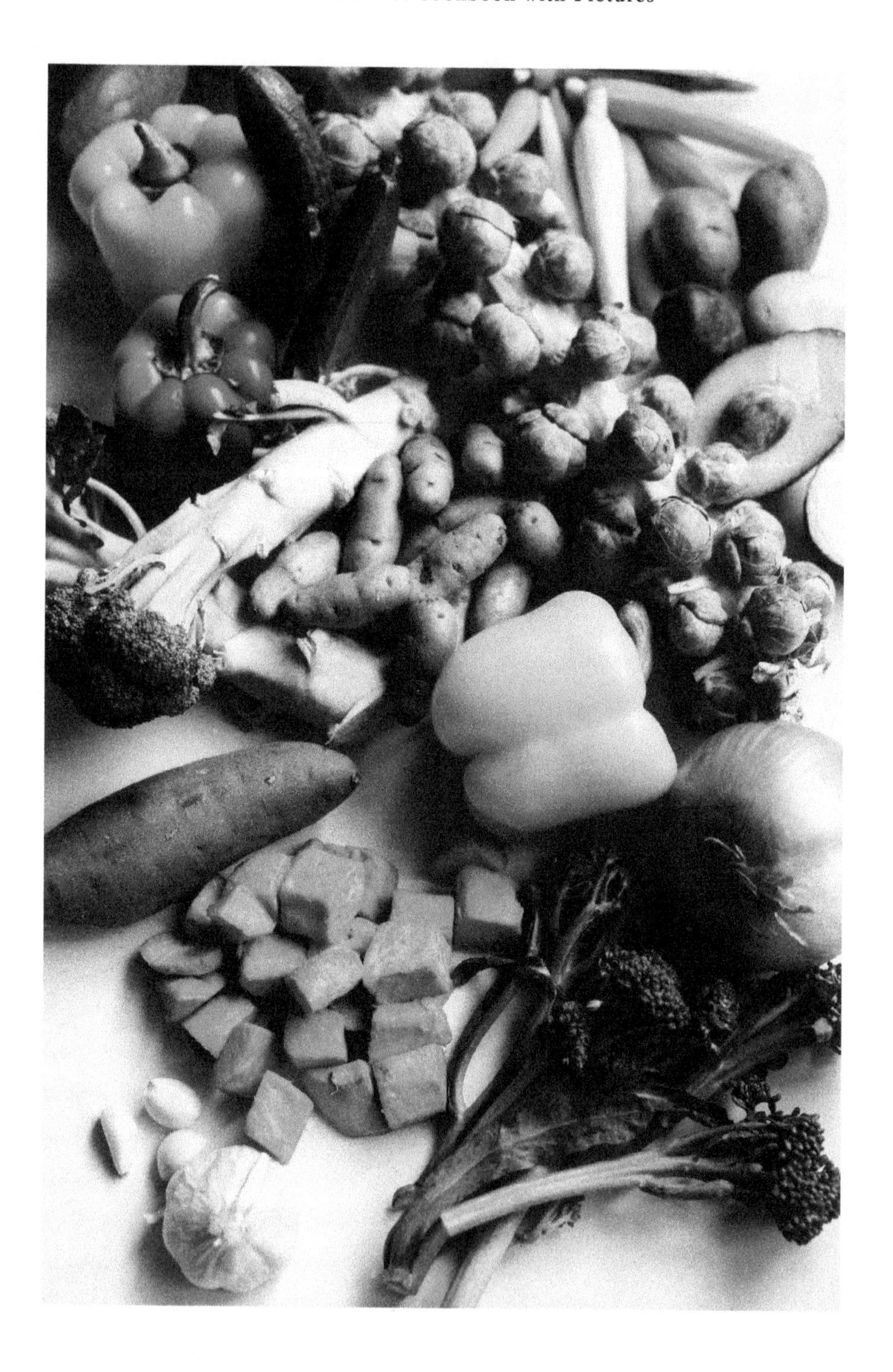

Introduction

As someone who was once in your shoes, I know that changing the way you eat can seem daunting. But keep in mind that this way of eating is not about what you can't eat; it's about all the delicious, nutritious foods you can eat. My goal with this book is to empower you to enjoy all the benefits of a whole-food, plant-based diet. So before we dive into the recipes, let's take a closer look at what exactly a whole-food, plant-based diet is and why it's so great.

Benefits of the Plant-Based Diet

When making the switch over to the plant-based eating plan, there are a number of benefits that come to mind. While these benefits are not immediate, they do manifest themselves in a relatively short period of time. As such, patience is an important key when looking to get the most out of this new dietary approach.

We are going to explore the benefits that come with the plant-based eating plan and how you can take full advantage of such benefits. Most importantly, you can find a great set of benefits which have the possibility of changing your life significantly.

Weight Loss

The most common reason why folks make this switch is for the purpose of losing weight. Truthfully, there is a great deal of logic in making this switch for the purpose of losing weight. Many individuals try their hardest to lose weight, yet they seem to come up short. And, while there are many factors that go into losing weight, the fact of the matter is that often there is a need to make a radical switch in eating habits.

The reasoning behind this lies in the functioning of the metabolism. The consumption of certain types of food, especially processed ones, creates a condition in which the body is unable to digest foods in the same manner.

For example, when you consume too much dairy, sugar and refined carbohydrates, your body quickly ships them off to fat storage. You would need to do massive amounts of exercise before you actually are able to tap into the body's fat reserves. Then, when you decide to cut down on the consumption of these foods, but not altogether, you end up causing your body to become confused.

To compound the issue, eating meat tends to slow down your metabolism as it takes much longer to digest meats, especially red meat, than it does to digest and process plant-based foods. As a result, you don't see the results you'd like to see.

When you switch over to the plant-based eating plan, you drastically alter your diet by cutting out the elements which slow down your metabolism. In return, your metabolism gets a break and progressively begins to speed up. In a manner of speaking, you are lightening the load on your metabolism as opposed to increasing it.

As your metabolism begins to speed up, you're able to digest foods faster and begin to accelerate the rate at which calories and nutrients are absorbed. Moreover, since plant-based foods don't accrue fat and calories like meat and processed foods do, then there is a definite advantage to boost weight loss. At the end of the day, consuming a great deal of plant-based foods makes a lot more sense if you're looking to lose weight.

Managing Illnesses

First, a bit of a disclaimer: if you are dealing with any medical condition, it is always a good idea to check with your doctor before making the switch. It might be that you have some type of dietary restriction that may interfere with the plant-based eating plan. While this is rather unusual, it's always a good idea to be sure you are not inadvertently putting yourself at risk. That being said, managing illnesses becomes a lot easier once you go on the plant-based eating plan. In short, the plant-based eating plan looks to maximize the nutrition that you get from the foods you consume. By taking away meats, especially processed ones, and substituting it for fresh fruits and vegetables, you're actually doing your body a favor by helping it recover and regenerate. However, there's one important secret that you might not be aware of. There are certain foods that we are allergic to, yet we don't even know how they are affecting us. In general, these are deep-fried, highly processed foods. In addition, sugary foods and drinks can do a number on your metabolism and immune system. The fact of the matter is that a lot of foods that we consume on a regular basis contain large amounts of oils and carbohydrates. These ingredients tend to cause inflammation in the body. Now, inflammation is a logical response to the body as it tries to isolate a damaged part. By isolating a part that has been hurt or at least the body thinks it's hurt, you cause all kinds of inflammation throughout your body. This causes the brain to release a series of hormones and chemicals that trigger a stress response in your body. This further complicates things are inflammation in your digestive tract will cause you to have trouble absorbing nutrients. In short, you're eating and feeling full, but you're not actually getting any nutrition. When this process occurs, you are essentially asking for trouble. By embracing the plant-based eating plan, you are giving your body the tools it needs to repair itself. By taking away potentially toxic elements, you're enabling your immune system to repair the body and thereby help alleviate some of the worse symptoms of whatever condition you may have. While going on this dietary approach is not going to cure what ails you, it will certainly help you manage the symptoms better and enable a better quality of life.

Muscle Growth and Fitness

One of the biggest concerns for athletes centers around the plant-based eating plan providing enough nutrients and protein, especially for demanding exercise routines. The short answer is that yes, the plant-based eating plan can provide athletes with all the nutrition they need. However, they need to do it the right way. Now, it should be noted that most athletes are concerned about loading on protein especially if they are looking to bulk up. This is particularly true in the case of bodybuilders. In such cases, it's best to consume an additional protein supplement that can help provide the necessary protein load for building muscle. However, beyond the rigorous requirements that bodybuilders have, regular folks and athletes need not be worried. The fact of the matter is that the plant-based eating plan provides ample room for protein so long as it's consumed on a regular basis. For instance, nuts provide a good deal of protein and healthy fats. Of course, we're not advocating that you must consume large amounts of nuts. Still, consuming a healthy dose will provide you with the building blocks you need. Moreover, all leafy greens, especially the dark greens, are packed with minerals that your body needs to maintain proper functioning. This is important when you consider the fact that the building blocks for the body are contained in the 90+ nutrients that are needed for a healthy body. These nutrients are found across a variety of plants. So, if you have a predominantly meat-based diet, you might be missing out on some of the most important nutrients that the body needs in order to keep fit and healthy.

Boosting the Immune System When on the Plant-Based Eating Plan and Through Supplementation

This is a legitimate question that comes up during this discussion. The fact of the matter is that we should all consume a vitamin and mineral supplement regardless of the type of diet we follow. It just makes sense to do so since the body needs a host of nutrients in order to function efficiently. As a result, a supplement helps fill the gaps that nutrition leaves behind.

While it's always a good idea to double-check with your doctor before taking any supplements, you can basically pick the supplement of your choice. It's a good idea to consume one that has a wide range of vitamins and minerals. These components help the body recover and regenerate many of the parts that get worn down over time. In some cases, chronic exposure to stress leaves considerable effects behind. Consequently, combining your new plant-based eating plan with a solid multivitamin and multimineral pack can help you get back on track.

Moreover, supplementation is a good idea when you have a demanding lifestyle, be it a result of physical exercise or working long hours. Please bear in mind that being able to put in a great deal of nutrients in your body will help it fight off common illnesses such as colds and the flu, while giving your immune system a fighting chance against any nasty bugs that might come your way.

Overall Health and Wellbeing

Most folks who make the switch over to the plant-based eating plan, describe feeling much "lighter" within the first few days. The reason for this is that your body begins an automatic detox program. By stopping the consumption of meat and other processed foods, you are allowing your body to get rid of these potentially toxic foods.

As your body begins to detox, your immune system, digestive tract, and metabolism all begin to function at a more efficient rate. The end result is a much lighter body. By "lighter" we mean that you are not carrying out as much potentially harmful substances as compared to the past.

To put this point into specific relief. When you are intoxicated by the foods you eat, it's quite common to feel a "full" stomach and experience bloating. This is a clear-cut sign that your body is going through an inflammatory process.

Can you stop this from happening?

Absolutely!

But you must focus on cutting out as much as you can of the processed foods you are eating in addition to meat. In fact, you will find that some folks in the health and fitness community go on "meat fasts" for short periods of time. What happens during this time is that a person will forego meat and animal products for a specific amount of time, say, a week or so. During this time, the intention is to help the body detox. When this happens, the resources the body has allocated to digesting meat are now assigned to other functions.

For instance, digesting meat requires a great deal of water. So, when you are digesting large amounts of meat, your body needs to consume lots of water just to flush out the meat you have eaten. This can leave you dehydrated. Consequently, you'll feel like you got run over by a train. When you stop eating as much meat or cut it out altogether, your body can now assign the water you consume to keeping your body hydrated. This is why many folks report higher levels of energy as compare to the past.

Is It Worth the Sacrifice?

Some folks look at switching over to a plant-based eating plan like a sacrifice. They feel like they are giving up on their favorite foods in favor of a healthier eating approach. The fact of the matter is that making this switch, even if it's just temporary, makes all the sense in the world. When you make this shift, your body will automatically begin to make the necessary adjustments.

The reality is that the downside to the plant-based eating plan is all in your head. You may think you lack the willpower to do it. Truthfully, you have it in you. All you need to do make a commitment to improving your overall health and wellbeing. When you begin to see the results, you won't want to go back.

Breakfasts

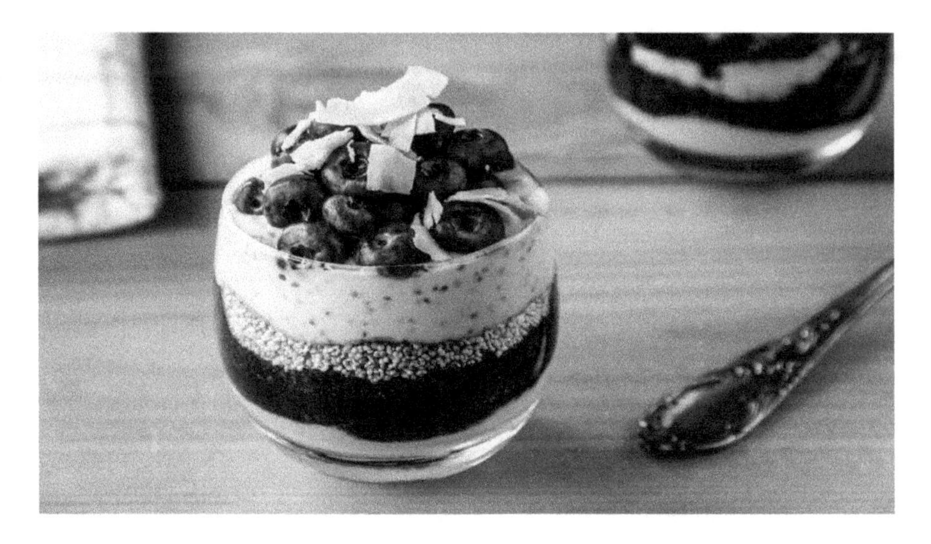

1. Breakfast Blueberry Muffins

Preparation Time: 15 minutes

Cooking Time: 25 minutes

Servings: 12

Ingredients:

Cooking spray

1 ½ cups rolled oats

¼ teaspoon baking soda

1 teaspoon baking powder

½ cup unsweetened applesauce

⅓ cup packed light brown sugar

¼ teaspoon salt

3 tablespoons vegetable oil

3 tablespoons water

1 tablespoon flax meal

1 teaspoon vanilla extract

¾ cup blueberries, sliced in half

Directions:

Preheat your oven to 350 degrees F.

Spray your muffin pan with oil.

Add the oats in a food processor.

Pulse until ground.

Stir in the rest of the ingredients except blueberries.

Pulse until smooth.

Pour the batter into the muffin pan.

Top with the blueberries.

Bake in the oven for 25 minutes.

Store in a glass jar with lid.

Nutrition: Calories: 106 fat: 4.6g Saturated fat: 0.4g Sodium: 118mg Potassium: 66mg Carbohydrates: 15.5g Fiber: 1.5g Sugar: 8g Protein: 1.5g

2. Oatmeal with Pears

Preparation Time: 15 minutes

Cooking Time: 15 minutes

Serving: 1

Ingredients:

¼ cup roll ed oats

¼ cup pear, sliced

1/8 teaspoon ground ginger

1/8 teaspoon ground cinnamon

Directions:

Cook the oats according to the directions in the package.

Stir in pear and ginger.

Sprinkle with cinnamon.

Store in a glass jar with lid.

Refrigerate overnight.

Nutrition: Calories: 108 fat: 2g Saturated fat: 0.1g Sodium: 5mg Potassium: 71mg Carbohydrates: 21g Fiber: 3g Sugar: 4g Protein: 3g

3. Yogurt with Cucumber

Preparation Time: 5 minutes

Cooking Time: 0 minute

Serving: 1

Ingredients:

1 cup soy yogurt

½ cucumber, diced

¼ teaspoon lemon zest

¼ teaspoon freshly squeezed lemon juice

Salt to taste

Chopped mint leaves

Directions:

Put all the ingredients in a glass jar with lid.

Refrigerate overnight or up to 2 days.

Nutrition: Calories: 164 fat: 3.9g Saturated fat: 2.5g Cholesterol: 15mg Sodium: 319mg Potassium: 683mg Carbohydrates: 19.1g Fiber: 0.6g Sugar: 18g Protein: 13.3g

4. Breakfast Casserole

Preparation Time: 20 minutes

Cooking Time: 43 minutes

Servings: 6

Ingredients:

10 oz. spinach

9 oz. artichoke hearts

2 cloves garlic, minced

¾ cup sun-dried tomatoes, chopped

½ teaspoon red pepper flakes

1 teaspoon lemon zest

1 tablespoon olive oil

2 cups almond milk

1 cup vegan cheese, crumbled

8 cups whole wheat bread, chopped

Directions:

Squeeze the spinach to release the liquid.

Add the spinach to a bowl.

Stir in the artichoke hearts.

In a pan over low heat, cook the garlic, tomatoes, red pepper and lemon zest in oil for 3 minutes.

Add the spinach and artichokes.

Remove from heat.

Transfer to a baking pan.

Stir in the spinach mixture and bread.

Let sit for 30 minutes.

Bake in the oven at 350 degrees F for 40 minutes.

Store in a food container and refrigerate.

Reheat before serving.

Nutrition: Calories: 277 fat: 9.9g Saturated fat: 4.5g Cholesterol: 136mg Sodium: 498mg Potassium: 542mg Carbohydrates: 30.5g Fiber: 4.8g Sugar: 6g Protein: 14.4g

5. Berries with Mascarpone on Toasted Bread

Preparation Time: 10 minutes   Cooking Time: 0 minute

Servings: 1

Ingredients:

1 slice whole-wheat bread

2 tablespoons mascarpone cheese

1/8 cup raspberries

1/8 cup strawberries

1 teaspoon fresh mint leaves

Directions:

Spread the cheese on the bread.

Top with the berries and chopped mint leaves.

Store in food container and refrigerate.

Toast in the oven when ready to eat.

Nutrition: Calories: 326 fat: 27.3g Saturated fat: 14.2g Cholesterol: 70mg Sodium: 130mg Potassium: 115mg Carbohydrates: 15.1g Fiber: 4.1g Sugar: 3g Protein: 7.9g

6. Fruit Cup

Preparation Time: 15 minutes Cooking Time: 0 minute Servings: 4

Ingredients:

2 cups melon, sliced

2 cups strawberries, sliced

2 cups grapes, sliced in half

2 cups peaches, sliced

3 tablespoons freshly squeezed lime juice

½ teaspoon ground ginger

1 tablespoon honey

3 teaspoons lime zest

¼ cup coconut flakes, toasted

Directions:

Toss the fruits in lime juice, ginger and honey. Sprinkle the lime zest on top.

Top with the coconut flakes.

Nutrition: Calories: 65 Total fat: 1.3g Saturated fat: 1.1g Sodium: 20mg Potassium: 247mg Carbohydrates: 13.9g Fiber: 1.6g Sugar: 10g Protein: 1g

7. Oatmeal with Black Beans & Cheddar

Preparation Time: 10 minutes

Cooking Time: 0 minute

Servings: 2

Ingredients:

½ cup rolled oats

¼ cup Vegan yogurt

½ cup almond milk

2 tablespoons seasoned black beans

2 tablespoons Cheddar cheese, shredded

1 stalk scallion, minced

1 tablespoon cilantro, chopped

Directions:

Mix all the ingredients except the cilantro in a glass jar with lid. Refrigerate for up to 5 days. Sprinkle the cilantro on top before serving.

Nutrition: Calories: 47 Total fat: 1.2g Saturated fat: 0.5g Sodium: 30mg Potassium: 151mg Carbohydrates: 11g Fiber: 1.9g Sugar: 9g Protein: 2g

8. Breakfast Smoothie

Preparation Time: 10 minutes

Cooking Time: 0 minute

Servings: 2

Ingredients:

½ cup strawberries

½ cup mango, sliced

½ banana, sliced

½ cup coconut milk

1 tablespoon cashew butter

1 tablespoon ground chia seeds

Directions:

Put all the ingredients in a blender.

Pulse until smooth.

Refrigerate overnight.

Nutrition: Calories: 299 Total fat: 14.5g Saturated fat: 4.2g Sodium: 64mg Potassium: 599mg Carbohydrates: 42.4g Fiber: 8.5g Sugar: 23g Protein: 5.3g

9. Yogurt with Beets & Raspberries

Preparation Time: 5 minutes

Cooking Time: 0 minute

Servings: 1

Ingredients:

1 cup soy yogurt

½ cup beets, cooked and sliced

1 tablespoon raspberry jam

1 tablespoon almonds, slivered

Directions:

Mix all the ingredients in a glass jar with lid.

Sprinkle the almonds on top.

Refrigerate for up to 2 days.

Nutrition: Calories: 281 Total fat: 7.3g Saturated fat: 2.7g Cholesterol: 15mg Sodium: 237mg Potassium: 882mg Carbohydrates: 40.2g Fiber: 2.5g Sugar: 36g Protein: 15.7g

10. Curry Oatmeal

Preparation Time: 10 minutes

Cooking Time: 0 minute

Servings: 3

Ingredients:

1 tablespoon pure peanut butter

½ cup rolled oats

½ cup coconut milk

½ teaspoon curry powder

1 teaspoon tamari

¼ cup cooked kale

1 tablespoon cilantro, chopped

2 tablespoons tomatoes, chopped

Directions:

Mix all the ingredients except the kale, cilantro and tomatoes.

Transfer to a glass jar with lid.

Refrigerate for up to 5 days.

Top with the remaining ingredients when ready to serve.

Nutrition: Calories: 307 Total fat: 13.8g Saturated fat: 4g Cholesterol: 12mg Sodium: 467mg Potassium: 890mg Carbohydrates: 34.1g Fiber: 3g Sugar: 2g Protein: 10.1g

11. Breakfast Cherry Delight

Preparation time: 10 minutes

Cooking time: 8 hours and 10 minutes

Servings: 4

Ingredients:

2 cups almond milk

2 cups water

1 cup steel cut oats

2 tablespoons cocoa powder

1/3 cup cherries, pitted

¼ Cup maple syrup

½ Teaspoon almond extract

For the sauce:

2 tablespoons water

1 and ½ cups cherries, pitted and chopped

¼ Teaspoon almond extract

Directions:

Put the almond milk in your slow cooker.

Add 2 cups water, oats, cocoa powder, 1/3 cup cherries, maples syrup and ½ teaspoon almond extract.

Stir, cover and cook on low for 8 hours.

In a small pan, mix 2 tablespoons water with 1 and ½ cups cherries and ¼ teaspoon almond extract, stir well, bring to a simmer over medium heat and cook for 10 minutes until it thickens.

Divide oatmeal into breakfast bowls, top with the cherries sauce and serve.

Enjoy!

Nutrition: calories 150, fat 1, fiber 2, carbs 6, protein 5

12. Crazy Maple and Pear Breakfast

Preparation time: 10 minutes

Cooking time: 9 hours

Servings: 2

Ingredients:

1 pear, cored and chopped

½ Teaspoon maple extract

2 cups coconut milk

½ Cup steel cut oats

½ Teaspoon vanilla extract

1 tablespoon stevia

¼ Cup walnuts, chopped for serving

Cooking spray

Directions:

Spray your slow cooker with some cooking spray and add coconut milk.

Also, add maple extract, oats, pear, stevia and vanilla extract, stir, cover and cook on low for 9 hours.

Stir your oatmeal again, divide it into breakfast bowls and serve with chopped walnuts on top.

Enjoy!

Nutrition: calories 150, fat 3, fiber 2, carbs 6, protein 6

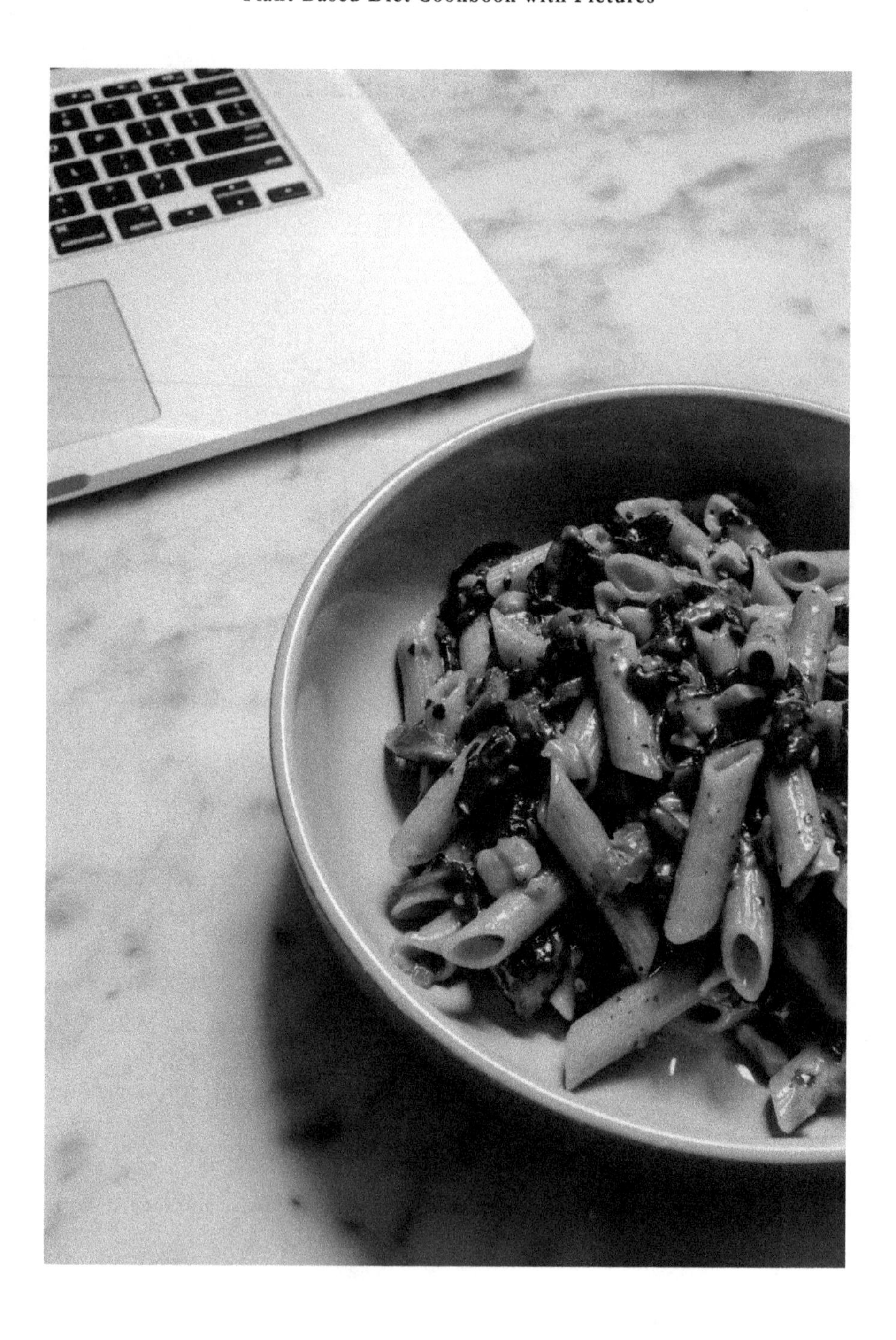

Entrées

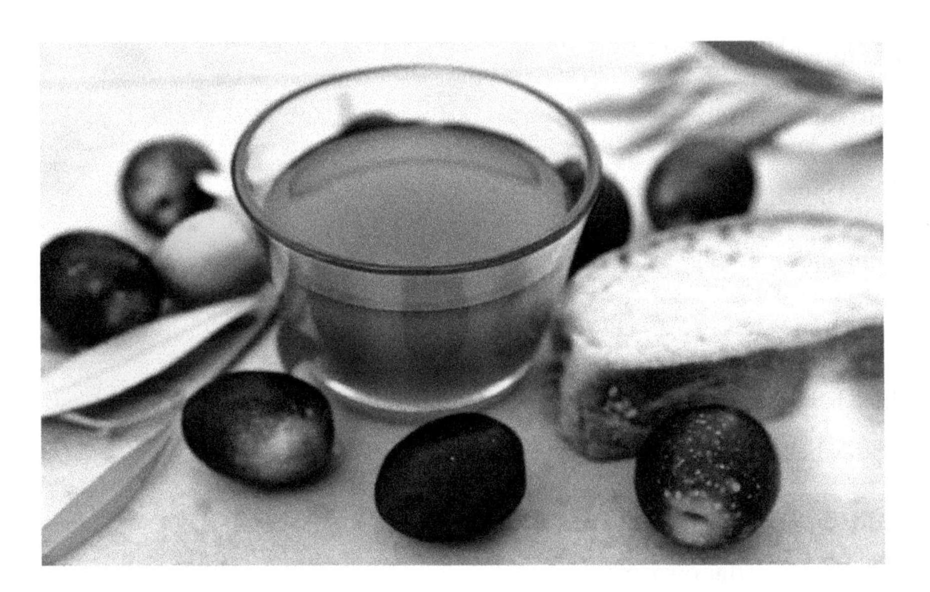

13. Black Bean Dip

Preparation time: 1 hour and 30 minutes

Cooking time: 1 hour

Servings: 10

Ingredients:

2 15-ounce cans black beans, rinsed and drained

1 jalapeno pepper, seeded and minced

½ of a red bell pepper, seeded and diced

½ of a yellow bell pepper, seeded and diced

½ of s small red onion, diced

1 cup fresh cilantro, finely chopped

Zest of 1 lime

Juice of 1 lime

1 10-ounce can Ro*tel, drained

½ teaspoon Kosher salt

¼ teaspoon ground black pepper

Directions:

In a large bowl, combine the garlic, green onions, beans, jalapeno, red and yellow bell pepper, onion, cilantro and mix together well.

Add the lime zest and juice, Ro-tel, salt and pepper and mix. Adjust seasoning to your own taste.

Refrigerate for at one hour, minimum, before serving, so the flavors have time to blend. Serve with wheat tortilla slices that have been crisped in the oven or with wheat or sesame crackers.

14. Cannellini Bean Cashew Dip

Preparation time: 1 hour

Cooking time: 1 hour

Servings: 8

Ingredients:

1 15-ounce can cannellini beans, rinsed and drained

½ cup raw cashews

1 clove garlic, smashed

2 tablespoons diced, red bell pepper

½ teaspoon sea salt

¼ teaspoon cayenne pepper

4 teaspoons lemon juice

2 tablespoons water

Dill sprigs or weed for garnish

Directions:

Place the beans, cashews, garlic and bell pepper in the food processor and pulse several times to break it up.

Add the salt, cayenne, lemon juice and water and process until smooth.

Scrape into a bowl, cover and refrigerate for at least an hour before serving.

Garnish with fresh dill and serve with vegetables, crackers or pita chips.

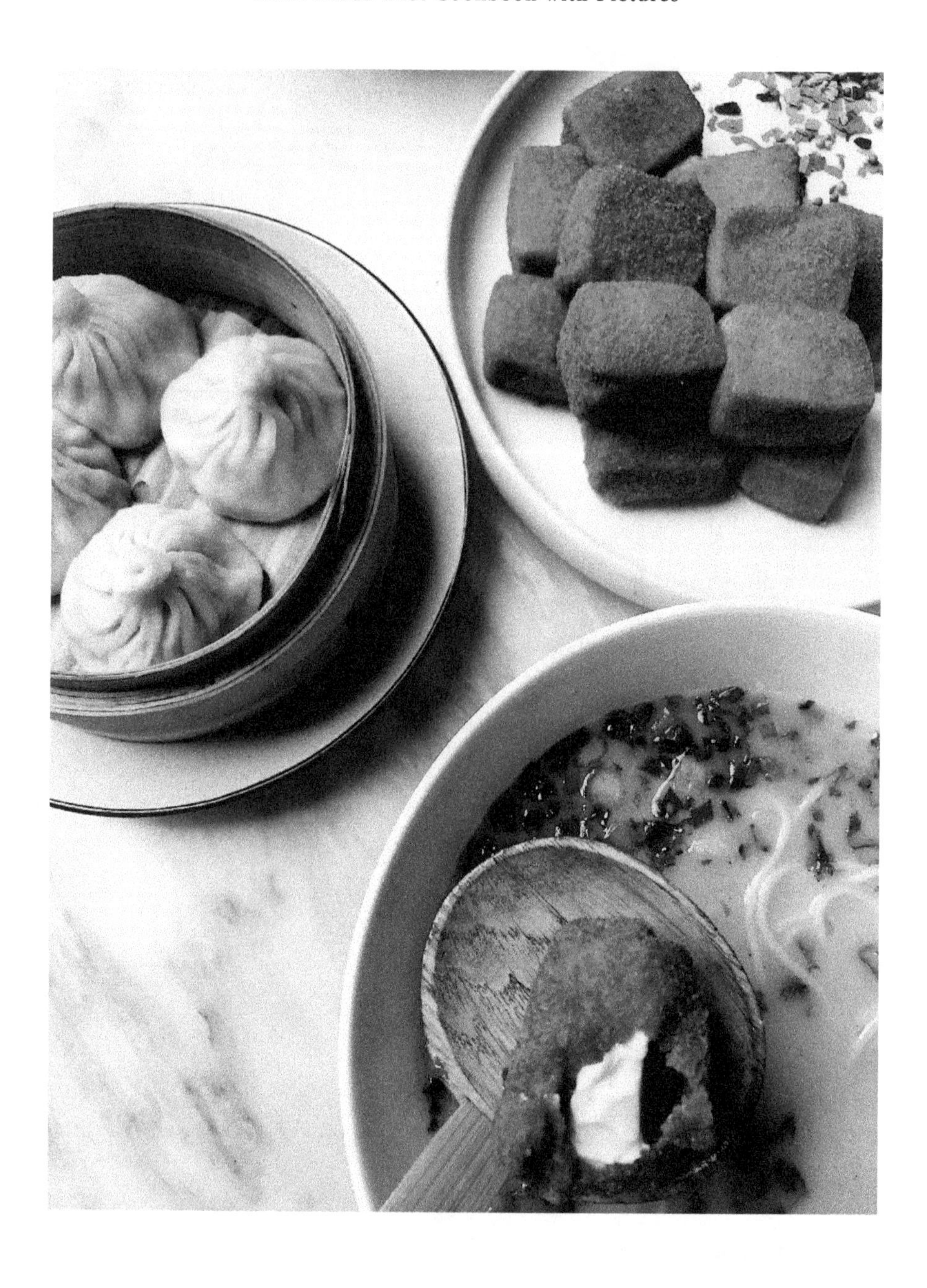

Soups, Salads, and Sides

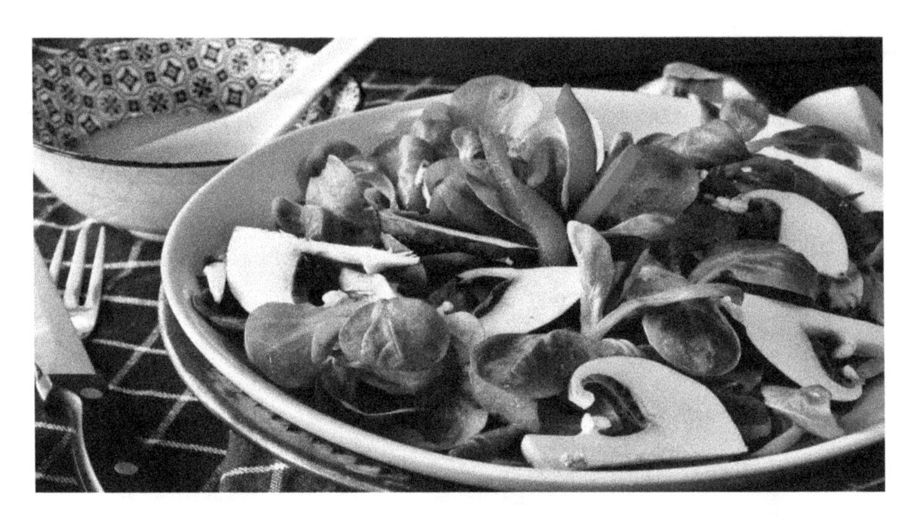

15. Spinach Soup with Dill and Basil

Preparation time: 10 minutes

Cooking time: 25 minutes

Servings: 8

Ingredients:

1 pound peeled and diced potatoes

1 tablespoon minced garlic

1 teaspoon dry mustard

6 cups vegetable broth

20 ounces chopped frozen spinach

2 cups chopped onion

1 ½ tablespoons salt

½ cup minced dill

1 cup basil

½ teaspoon ground black pepper

Directions:

Whisk onion, garlic, potatoes, broth, mustard, and salt in a pand cook it over medium flame. When it starts boiling, low down the heat and cover it with the lid and cook for 20 minutes. Add the remaining ingredients in it and blend it and cook it for few more minutes and serve it.

Nutrition: Carbohydrates 12g, protein 13g, fats 1g, calories 165.

16. Coconut Watercress Soup

Preparation time: 10 minutes

Cooking time: 20 minutes

Servings: 4

Ingredients:

1 teaspoon coconut oil

1 onion, diced

¾ cup coconut milk

Directions:

Preparing the ingredients.

Melt the coconut oil in a large pot over medium-high heat. Add the onion and cook until soft, about 5 minutes, then add the peas and the water. Bring to a boil, then lower the heat and add the watercress, mint, salt, and pepper.

Cover and simmer for 5 minutes. Stir in the coconut milk, and purée the soup until smooth in a blender or with an immersion blender.

Try this soup with any other fresh, leafy green—anything from spinach to collard greens to arugula to swiss chard.

Nutrition: calories: 178; protein: 6g; total fat: 10g; carbohydrates: 18g; fiber: 5g

17. Roasted Red Pepper and Butternut Squash Soup

Preparation time: 10 minutes

Cooking time: 45 minutes

Servings: 6

Ingredients:

1 small butternut squash

1 tablespoon olive oil

1 teaspoon sea salt

2 red bell peppers

1 yellow onion

1 head garlic

2 cups water, or vegetable broth

Zest and juice of 1 lime

1 to 2 tablespoons tahini

Pinch cayenne pepper

½ teaspoon ground coriander

½ teaspoon ground cumin

Toasted squash seeds (optional)

Directions:

Preparing the ingredients.

Preheat the oven to 350°f.

Prepare the squash for roasting by cutting it in half lengthwise, scooping out the seeds, and poking some holes in the flesh with a fork. Reserve the seeds if desired.

Rub a small amount of oil over the flesh and skin, then rub with a bit of sea salt and put the halves skin-side down in a large baking dish. Put it in the oven while you prepare the rest of the vegetables.

Prepare the peppers the exact same way, except they do not need to be poked.

Slice the onion in half and rub oil on the exposed faces. Slice the top off the head of garlic and rub oil on the exposed flesh.

After the squash has cooked for 20 minutes, add the peppers, onion, and garlic, and roast for another 20 minutes. Optionally, you can toast the squash seeds by putting them in the oven in a separate baking dish 10 to 15 minutes before the vegetables are finished.

Keep a close eye on them. When the vegetables are cooked, take them out and let them cool before handling them. The squash will be very soft when poked with a fork.

Scoop the flesh out of the squash skin into a large pot (if you have an immersion blender) or into a blender.

Chop the pepper roughly, remove the onion skin and chop the onion roughly, and squeeze the garlic cloves out of the head, all into the pot or blender. Add the water, the lime zest and juice, and the tahini. Purée the soup, adding more water if you like, to your desired consistency. Season with the salt, cayenne, coriander, and cumin. Serve garnished with toasted squash seeds (if using).

Nutrition: calories: 156; protein: 4g; total fat: 7g; saturated fat: 11g; carbohydrates: 22g; fiber: 5g

18. Tomato Pumpkin Soup

Preparation time: 25 minutes Cooking time: 15 minutes

Servings: 4

Ingredients:

2 cups pumpkin, diced

1/2 cup tomato, chopped

1/2 cup onion, chopped

1 1/2 tsp curry powder

1/2 tsp paprika

2 cups vegetable stock

1 tsp olive oil

1/2 tsp garlic, minced

Directions:

In a saucepan, add oil, garlic, and onion and sauté for 3 minutes over medium heat.

Add remaining ingredients into the saucepan and bring to boil.

Reduce heat and cover and simmer for 10 minutes.

Puree the soup using a blender until smooth.

Stir well and serve warm.

Nutrition: calories 70; fat 2.7 g; carbohydrates 13.8 g; sugar 6.3 g; protein 1.9 g; cholesterol 0 mg

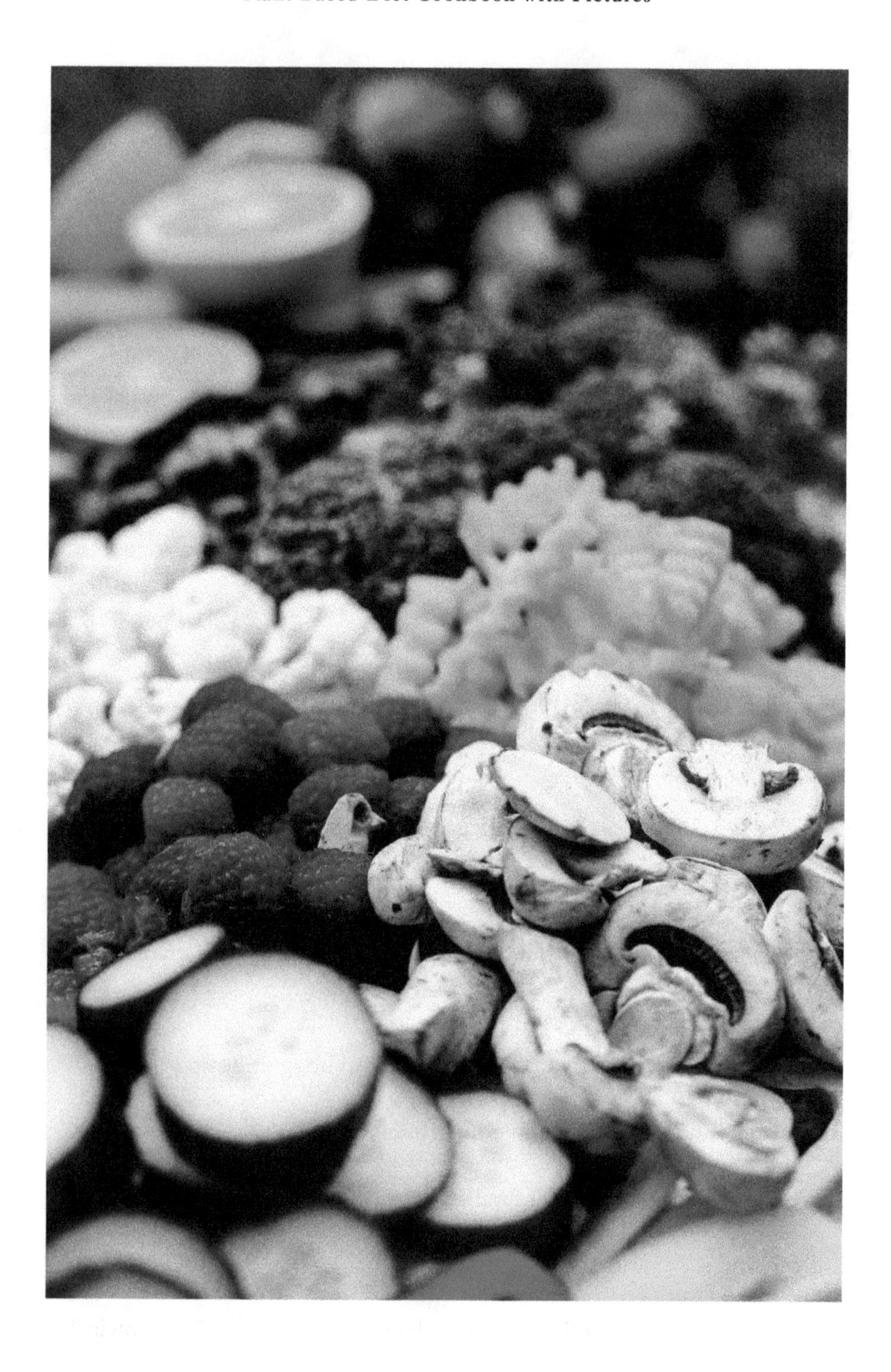

Lunch Recipes

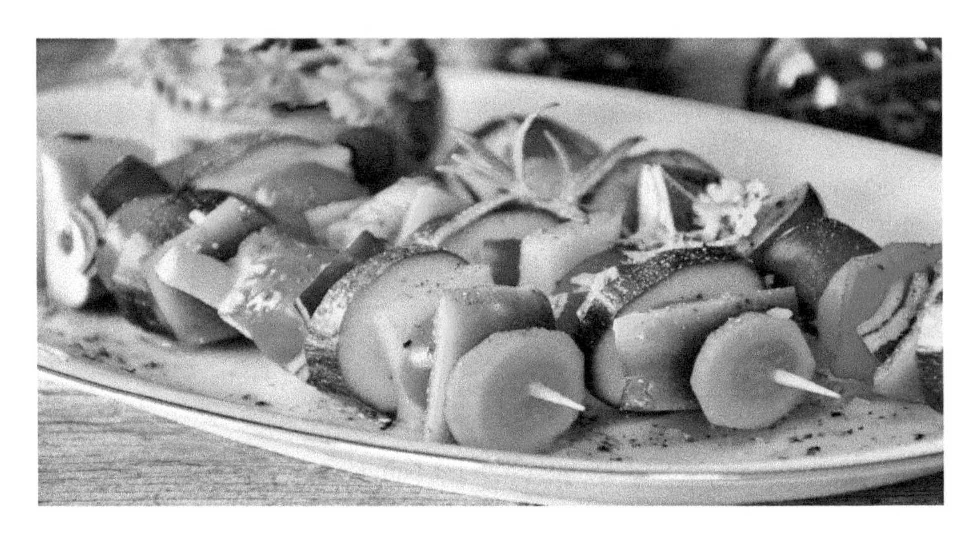

19. Cauliflower Latke

Preparation Time: 15 minutes

Cooking Time: 30 minutes

Servings: 4

Ingredients:

12 oz. cauliflower rice, cooked

1 egg, beaten

1/3 cup cornstarch

Salt and pepper to taste

¼ cup vegetable oil, divided

Chopped onion chives

Direction

Squeeze excess water from the cauliflower rice using paper towels.

Place the cauliflower rice in a bowl.

Stir in the egg and cornstarch.

Season with salt and pepper.

Pour 2 tablespoons of oil into a pan over medium heat.

Add 2 to 3 tablespoons of the cauliflower mixture into the pan.

Cook for 3 minutes per side or until golden.

Repeat until you've used up the rest of the batter.

Garnish with chopped chives.

Nutrition: Calories: 209 Total fat: 15.2g Saturated fat: 1.4g Cholesterol: 47mg Sodium: 331mg Potassium: 21mg Carbohydrates: 13.4g Fiber: 1.9g Sugar: 2g Protein: 3.4g

20. Roasted Brussels Sprouts

Preparation Time: 30 minutes Cooking Time: 20 minutes

Servings: 4

Ingredients:

1 lb. Brussels sprouts, sliced in half

1 shallot, chopped

1 tablespoon olive oil

Salt and pepper to taste

2 teaspoons balsamic vinegar

¼ cup pomegranate seeds

¼ cup goat cheese, crumbled

Direction:

Preheat your oven to 400 degrees F. Coat the Brussels sprouts with oil.

Sprinkle with salt and pepper.

Transfer to a baking pan.

Roast in the oven for 20 minutes.

Drizzle with the vinegar.

Sprinkle with the seeds and cheese before serving.

Nutrition: Calories: 117 Total fat: 5.7g Saturated fat: 1.8g Cholesterol: 4mg Sodium: 216mg Potassium: 491mg Carbohydrates: 13.6g Fiber: 4.8g Sugar: 5g Protein: 5.8g

21. Brussels Sprouts & Cranberries Salad

Preparation Time: 10 minutes

Cooking Time: 0 minute

Servings: 6

Ingredients:

3 tablespoons lemon juice

¼ cup olive oil

Salt and pepper to taste

1 lb. Brussels sprouts, sliced thinly

¼ cup dried cranberries, chopped

½ cup pecans, toasted and chopped

½ cup vegan parmesan cheese, shaved

Direction

Mix the lemon juice, olive oil, salt and pepper in a bowl.

Toss the Brussels sprouts, cranberries and pecans in this mixture.

Sprinkle the Parmesan cheese on top.

Nutrition: Calories 245 Total Fat 18.9 g Saturated Fat 9 g Cholesterol 3 mg Sodium 350 mg Total Carbohydrate 15.9 g Dietary Fiber 5 g Protein 6.4 g Total Sugars 10 g Potassium 20 mg

22. Potato Latke

Preparation Time: 15 minutes

Cooking Time: 10 minutes

Servings: 6

Ingredients:

3 eggs, beaten

1 onion, grated

1 ½ teaspoons baking powder

Salt and pepper to taste

2 lb. potatoes, peeled and grated

¼ cup all-purpose flour

4 tablespoons vegetable oil

Chopped onion chives

Direction

Preheat your oven to 400 degrees F.

In a bowl, beat the eggs, onion, baking powder, salt and pepper.

Squeeze moisture from the shredded potatoes using paper towel.

Add potatoes to the egg mixture.

Stir in the flour.

Pour the oil into a pan over medium heat.

Cook a small amount of the batter for 3 to 4 minutes per side.

Repeat until the rest of the batter is used.

Garnish with the chives.

Nutrition: Calories: 266 Total fat: 11.6g Saturated fat: 2g Cholesterol: 93mg Sodium: 360mg Potassium: 752mg Carbohydrates: 34.6g Fiber: 9g Sugar: 3g Protein: 7.5g

23. Broccoli Rabe

Preparation Time: 15 minutes Cooking Time: 15 minutes

Servings: 8

Ingredients:

2 oranges, sliced in half

1 lb. broccoli rabe

2 tablespoons sesame oil, toasted

Salt and pepper to taste

1 tablespoon sesame seeds, toasted

Direction

Pour the oil into a pan over medium heat.

Add the oranges and cook until caramelized.

Transfer to a plate.

Put the broccoli in the pan and cook for 8 minutes.

Squeeze the oranges to release juice in a bowl.

Stir in the oil, salt and pepper.

Coat the broccoli rabe with the mixture.

Sprinkle seeds on top.

Nutrition: Calories: 59 Total fat: 4.4g Saturated fat: 0.6g Sodium: 164mg Potassium: 160mg Carbohydrates: 4.1g Fiber: 1.6g Sugar: 2g Protein: 2.2g

24. Whipped Potatoes

Preparation Time: 20 minutes

Cooking Time: 35 minutes

Servings: 10

Ingredients:

4 cups water

3 lb. potatoes, sliced into cubes

3 cloves garlic, crushed

6 tablespoons vegan butter

2 bay leaves

10 sage leaves

½ cup Vegan yogurt

¼ cup low-fat milk

Salt to taste

Direction

Boil the potatoes in water for 30 minutes or until tender.

Drain.

In a pan over medium heat, cook the garlic in butter for 1 minute.

Add the sage and cook for 5 more minutes.

Discard the garlic.

Use a fork to mash the potatoes.

Whip using an electric mixer while gradually adding the butter, yogurt, and milk.

Season with salt.

Nutrition: Calories: 169 Total fat: 7.6g Saturated fat: 4.7g Cholesterol: 21mg Sodium: 251mg Potassium: 519mg Carbohydrates: 22.1g Fiber: 1.5g Sugar: 2g Protein: 4.2g

25. Quinoa Avocado Salad

Preparation Time: 15 minutes

Cooking Time: 4 minutes

Servings: 4

Ingredients:

2 tablespoons balsamic vinegar

¼ cup cream

¼ cup buttermilk

5 tablespoons freshly squeezed lemon juice, divided

1 clove garlic, grated

2 tablespoons shallot, minced

Salt and pepper to taste

2 tablespoons avocado oil, divided

1 ¼ cups quinoa, cooked

2 heads endive, sliced

2 firm pears, sliced thinly

2 avocados, sliced

¼ cup fresh dill, chopped

Direction

Combine the vinegar, cream, milk, 1 tablespoon lemon juice, garlic, shallot, salt and pepper in a bowl.

Pour 1 tablespoon oil into a pan over medium heat.

Heat the quinoa for 4 minutes.

Transfer quinoa to a plate.

Toss the endive and pears in a mixture of remaining oil, remaining lemon juice, salt and pepper.

Transfer to a plate.

Toss the avocado in the reserved dressing.

Add to the plate.

Top with the dill and quinoa.

Nutrition: Calories: 431 Total fat: 28.5g Saturated fat: 8g Cholesterol: 13mg Sodium: 345mg Potassium: 779mg Carbohydrates: 42.7g Fiber: 6g Sugar: 3g Protein: 6.6g

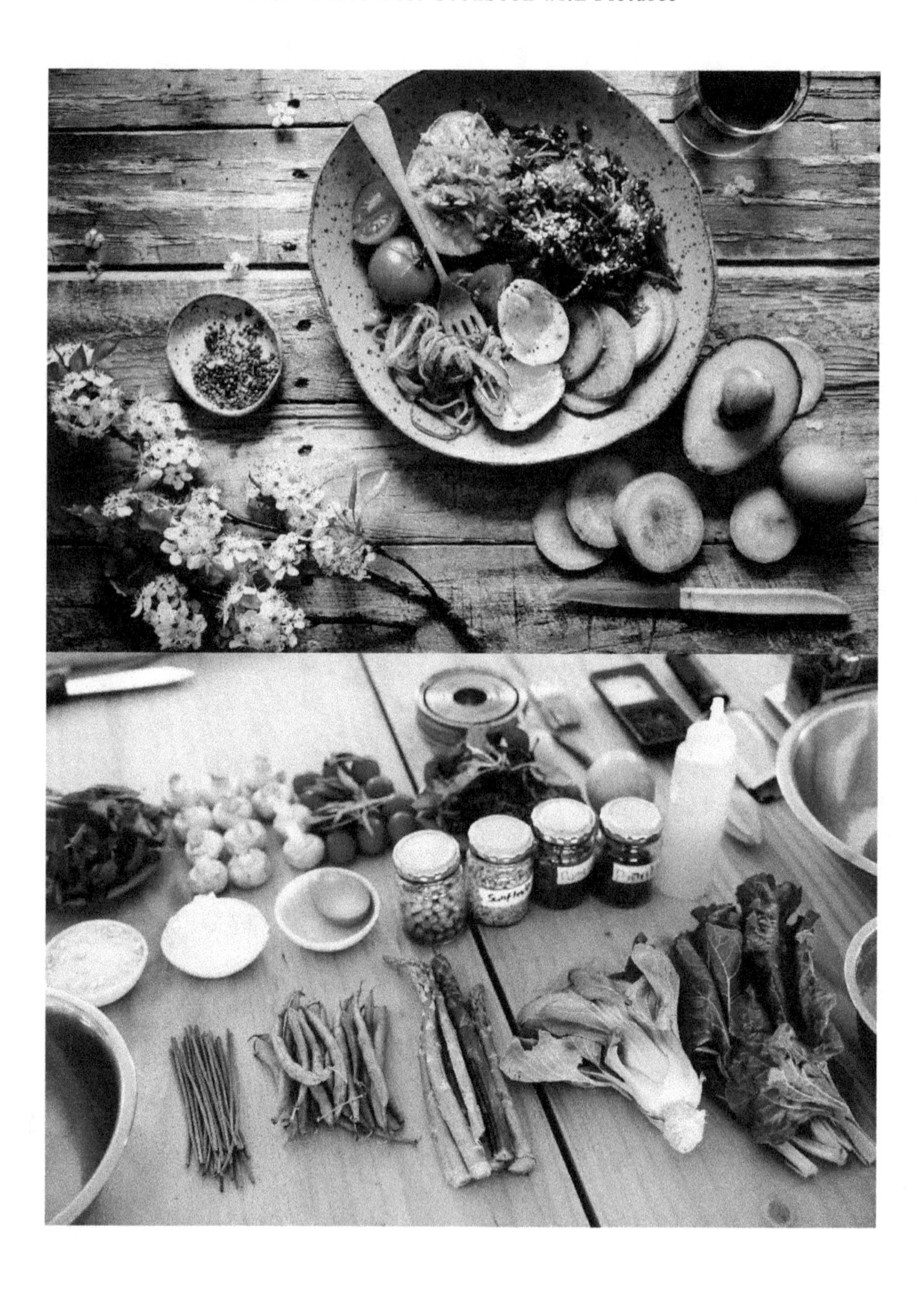

Dinner Recipes

26. Broccoli & black beans stir fry

Preparation time 60 minutes

Cooking time: 10 minutes

Servings: 6

Ingredients:

4 cups broccoli flore ts

2 cups cooked black beans

1 tablespoon sesame oil

4 teaspoons sesame seeds

2 cloves garlic, finely minced

2 teaspoons ginger, finely chopped

A large pinch red chili flakes

A pinch turmeric powder

Salt to taste

Lime juice to taste (optional)

Direction:

Steam broccoli for 6 minutes. Drain and set aside.

Warm the sesame oil in a large frying pan over medium heat. Add sesame seeds, chili flakes, ginger, garlic, turmeric powder, and salt. Sauté for a couple of minutes.

Add broccoli and black beans and sauté until thoroughly heated.

Sprinkle lime juice and serve hot.

27. Stuffed peppers

Preparation time 40 minutes

Cooking time: 15 minutes

Servings: 8

Ingredients:

2 cans (15 ounces each) black beans, drained, rinsed

2 cups tofu, pressed, crumbled

3/4 cup green onion s, thinly sliced

1/2 cup fresh cilantro, chopped

1/4 cup vegetable oil

1/4 cup lime juice

3 cloves garlic, finely chopped

1/2 teaspoon salt

1/2 teaspoon chili powder

8 large bell peppers, halved lengthwise, deseeded

3 roma tomatoes, diced

Direction:

Mix together in a bowl all the ingredients except the bell peppers to make the filling.

Fill the peppers with this mixture.

Cut 8 aluminum foils of size 18 x 12 inches. Place 2 halves on each aluminum foil. Seal the peppers such that there is a gap on the sides.

Grill under direct heat for about 15 minutes.

Sprinkle with some cilantro and serve.

Recipes For Main Courses And Single Dishes

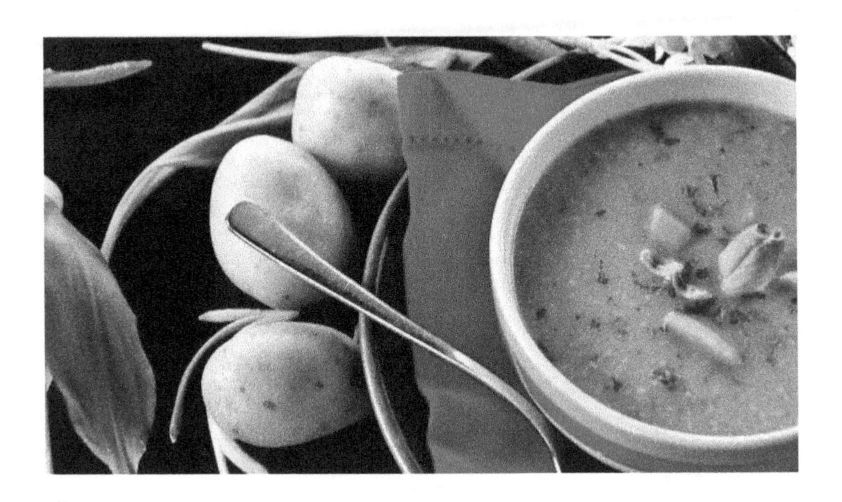

28. Noodles Alfredo with Herby Tofu

Preparation Time: 10 minutes

Cooking Time: 5 minutes

Servings: 4

Ingredients:

2 tbsp vegetable oil

2 (14 oz.) blocks extra-firm tofu, pressed and cubed

12 ounces eggless noodles

1 tbsp dried mixed herbs

2 cups cashews, soaked overnight and drained

¾ cups unsweetened almond milk

½ cup nutritional yeast

4 garlic cloves, roasted (roasting is optional but highly recommended)

½ cup onion, coarsely chopped

1 lemon, juiced

½ cup sun-dried tomatoes

Salt and black pepper to taste

2 tbsp chopped fresh basil leaves to garnish

Directions:

Heat the vegetable oil in a large skillet over medium heat.

Season the tofu with the mixed herbs, salt, black pepper, and fry in the oil until golden brown. Transfer to a paper-towel-lined plate and set aside. Turn the heat off.

In a blender, combine the almond milk, nutritional yeast, garlic, onion, and lemon juice. Set aside.

Reheat the vegetable oil in the skillet over medium heat and sauté the noodles for 2 minutes. Stir in the sundried tomatoes and the cashew (Alfredo) sauce. Reduce the heat to low and cook for 2 more minutes.

If the sauce is too thick, thin with some more almond milk to your desired thickness.

Dish the food, garnish with the basil and serve warm.

29. Lemon Couscous with Tempeh Kabobs

Preparation Time: 2 hours 15 minutes

Cooking Time: 2 hours

Servings: 4

Ingredients:

For the tempeh kabobs:

1 ½ cups of water

10 oz. tempeh, cut into 1-inch chunks

1 red onion, cut into 1-inch chunks

1 small yellow squash, cut into 1-inch chunks

1 small green squash, cut into 1-inch chunks

2 tbsp. olive oil

1 cup sugar-free barbecue sauce

8 wooden skewers, soaked

For the lemon couscous:

1 ½ cups whole wheat couscous

2 cups of water

Salt to taste

¼ cup chopped parsley

¼ chopped mint leaves

¼ cup chopped cilantro

1 lemon, juiced

1 medium avocado, pitted, sliced and peeled

Directions:

For the tempeh kabobs:

Boil the water in a medium pot over medium heat.

Once boiled, turn the heat off, and put the tempeh in it. Cover the lid and let the tempeh steam for 5 minutes (this is to remove its bitterness). Drain the tempeh after.

After, pour the barbecue sauce into a medium bowl, add the tempeh, and coat well with the sauce. Cover the bowl with plastic wrap and marinate for 2 hours. After 2 hours, preheat a grill to 350 F. On the skewers, alternately thread single chunks of the tempeh, onion, yellow squash, and green squash until the ingredients are exhausted.

Lightly grease the grill grates with olive oil, place the skewers on top and brush with some barbecue sauce. Cook for 3 minutes on each side while brushing with more barbecue sauce as you turn the kabobs.

Transfer to a plate for serving. For the lemon couscous: Meanwhile, as the kabobs cooked, pour the couscous, water, and salt into a medium bowl and steam in the microwave for 3 to 4 minutes. Remove the bowl from the microwave and allow slight cooling.

Stir in the parsley, mint leaves, cilantro, and lemon juice.

Garnish the couscous with the avocado slices and serve with the tempeh kabobs.

Smoothies, Snacks and Desserts

30. Chocolate Smoothie

Preparation Time: 5 min.

Cooking Time: 5 min.

Servings: 2

Ingredients:

¼ c. almond butter

¼ c. cocoa powder, unsweetened

½ c. coconut milk, canned

1 c. almond milk, unsweetened

Directions:

Before making the smoothie, freeze the almond milk into cubes using an ice cube tray. This would take a few hours, so prepare it ahead.

Blend everything using your preferred machine until it reaches your desired thickness.

Serve immediately and enjoy!

Nutrition: Calories: 147 | Carbohydrates: 8.2 g | Proteins: 4 g | Fats: 13.4 g

31. Chocolate Mint Smoothie

Preparation Time: 5 min.

Cooking Time: 5 min.

Serving: 1

Ingredients:

2 tbsp. sweetener of your choice

2 drops mint extract

1 tbsp. cocoa powder

½ avocado, medium

¼ c. coconut milk

1 c. almond milk, unsweetened

Directions:

In a high-speed blender, add all the ingredients and blend until smooth.

Add two to four ice cubes and blend.

Serve immediately and enjoy!

Nutrition: Calories: 401 | Carbohydrates: 6.3 g | Proteins: 5 g | Fats: 40.3 g

32. Cinnamon Roll Smoothie

Preparation Time: 2 min.

Cooking Time: 2 min.

Serving: 1

Ingredients:

1 t. cinnamon

1 scoop vanilla protein powder

½ c. of the following:

- almond milk, unsweetened
- coconut milk

Sweetener of your choice

Directions:

In a high-speed blender, add all the ingredients and blend.

Add two to four ice cubes and blend until smooth.

Serve immediately and enjoy!

Nutrition: Calories: 507 | Carbohydrates: 17 g | Proteins: 33.3 g | Fats: 34.9 g

33. Coconut Smoothie

Preparation Time: 2 min.

Cooking Time: 2 min.

Servings: 2

Ingredients:

1 t. chia seeds

1/8 c. almonds, soaked

1 c. coconut milk

1 avocado

Directions:

In a high-speed blender, add all the ingredients and blend until smooth.

Add your desired number of ice cubes, depending on your favored consistency, of course, and blend again.

Serve immediately and enjoy!

Nutrition: Calories: 584 | Carbohydrates: 22.5 g | Proteins: 8.3 g | Fats: 55.5g

34. Maca Almond Smoothie

Preparation Time: 5 min.

Cooking Time: 5 min.

Servings: 2

Ingredients:

½ t. vanilla extract

1 scoop maca powder

1 tbsp. almond butter

1 c. almond milk, unsweetened

2 avocados

Directions:

In a high-speed blender, add all the ingredients and blend until smooth.

Serve immediately and enjoy!

Nutrition: Calories: 758 | Carbohydrates: 28.6 g | Proteins: 9.3 g | Fats: 72.3 g

35. Blueberry Smoothie

Preparation Time: 5 min.

Cooking Time: 5 min.

Serving: 1

Ingredients:

¼ c. pumpkin seeds shelled unsalted

3 c. blueberries, frozen

2 avocados, peeled and halved

1 c. almond milk

Directions:

In a high-speed blender, add all the ingredients and blend until smooth.

Add two to four ice cubes and blend until smooth.

Serve immediately and enjoy!

Nutrition: Calories: 401 | Carbohydrates: 6.3 g | Proteins: 5 g | Fats: 40.3 g

36. Nutty Protein Shake

Preparation Time: 5 min.

Cooking Time: 5 min.

Serving: 1

Ingredients:

¼ avocado

2 tbsp. powdered peanut butter

1 tbsp. of the following:

- Cocoa powder
- Peanut butter

1 scoop protein powder

½ c. almond milk

Directions:

In a high-speed blender, add all the ingredients and blend until smooth.

Add two to four ice cubes and blend again.

Serve immediately and enjoy!

Nutrition: Calories: 694 | Carbohydrates: 30.8 g | Proteins: 40.8 g | Fats: 52 g

37. Cinnamon Pear Smoothie

Preparation Time: 2 min.

Cooking Time: 2 min.

Serving: 1

Ingredients:

1 t. cinnamon

1 scoop vanilla protein powder

½ c. of the following:

Almond milk, unsweetened

Coconut Milk

2 pears, cores removed

Sweetener of your choice

Directions:

In a high-speed blender, add all the ingredients and blend.

Add two or more ice cubes and blend again.

Serve immediately and enjoy!

Nutrition: Calories: 653 | Carbohydrates: 75.2 g | Proteins: 28.4 g | Fats: 32.2 g

38. Vanilla Milkshake

Preparation Time: 5 min.

Cooking Time: 5 min.

Servings: 4

Ingredients:

2 c. ice cubes

2 t. vanilla extract

6 tbsp. powdered erythritol

1 c. cream of dairy-free

½ c. coconut milk

Directions:

In a high-speed blender, add all the ingredients and blend.

Add ice cubes and blend until smooth.

Serve immediately and enjoy!

Nutrition: Calories: 125 | Carbohydrates: 6.8 g | Proteins: 1.2 g | Fats: 11.5 g

39. Raspberry Protein Shake

Preparation Time: 5 min.

Cooking Time: 5 min.

Serving: 1

Ingredients:

¼ avocado

1 c. raspberries, frozen

1 scoop protein powder

½ c. almond milk

Ice cubes

Directions:

In a high-speed blender add all the ingredients and blend until lumps of fruit disappear.

Add two to four ice cubes and blend to your desired consistency.

Serve immediately and enjoy!

Nutrition: Calories: 756 | Carbohydrates: 80.1 g | Proteins: 27.6 g | Fats: 40.7 g

40. Raspberry Almond Smoothie

Preparation Time: 5 min.

Cooking Time: 5 min.

Serving: 1

Ingredients:

10 Almonds, finely chopped

3 tbsp. almond butter

1 c. almond milk

1 c. Raspberries, frozen

Directions:

In a high-speed blender, add all the ingredients and blend until smooth.

Serve immediately and enjoy!

Nutrition: Calories: 449 | Carbohydrates: 26 g | Proteins: 14 g | Fats: 35 g

41. Apple Raspberry Cobbler

Preparation Time: 50 minutes

Servings: 4

A safer type of fruit cobbler where a cut in sugar enhances the fruit.

Ingredients

3 apples, peeled, cored, and chopped

2 tbsp pure date sugar

1 cup fresh raspberries

2 tbsp unsalted plant butter

½ cup whole-wheat flour

1 cup toasted rolled oats

2 tbsp pure date sugar

1 tsp cinnamon powder

Directions

Preheat the oven to 350 F and grease a baking dish with some plant butter.

Add the apples, date sugar, and 3 tbsp of water to a medium pot. Cook over low heat until the date sugar melts and then, mix in the raspberries. Cook until the fruits soften, 10 minutes.

Pour and spread the fruit mixture into the baking dish and set aside.

In a blender, add the plant butter, flour, oats, date sugar, and cinnamon powder. Pulse a few times until crumbly.

Spoon and spread the mixture on the fruit mix until evenly layered.

Bake in the oven for 25 to 30 minutes or until golden brown on top.

Remove the dessert, allow cooling for 2 minutes, and serve.

Nutritional info per serving

Calories 539 | Fats 12g| Carbs 105.7g | Protein 8.2g

42. White Chocolate Pudding

Preparation Time: 4 hours 20 minutes

Servings: 4

Ingredients

3 tbsp flax seed + 9 tbsp water

3 tbsp cornstarch

¼ tbsp salt

1 cup cashew cream

2 ½ cups almond milk

½ pure date sugar

1 tbsp vanilla caviar

6 oz unsweetened white chocolate chips

Whipped coconut cream for topping

Sliced bananas and raspberries for topping

Directions

In a small bowl, mix the flax seed powder with water and allow thickening for 5 minutes to make the flax egg.

In a large bowl, whisk the cornstarch and salt, and then slowly mix in the in the cashew cream until smooth. Whisk in the flax egg until well combined.

Pour the almond milk into a pot and whisk in the date sugar. Cook over medium heat while frequently stirring until the sugar dissolves. Reduce the heat to low and simmer until steamy and bubbly around the edges.

Pour half of the almond milk mixture into the flax egg mix, whisk well and pour this mixture into the remaining milk content in the pot. Whisk continuously until well combined.

Bring the new mixture to a boil over medium heat while still frequently stirring and scraping all the corners of the pot, 2 minutes.

Turn the heat off, stir in the vanilla caviar, then the white chocolate chips until melted. Spoon the mixture into a bowl, allow cooling for 2 minutes, cover with plastic wraps making sure to press the plastic onto the surface of the pudding, and refrigerate for 4 hours.

Remove the pudding from the fridge, take off the plastic wrap and whip for about a minute.

Spoon the dessert into serving cups, swirl some coconut whipping cream on top, and top with the bananas and raspberries. Enjoy immediately.

Nutritional info per serving

Calories 654 | Fats 47.9g| Carbs 52.1g | Protein 7.3g

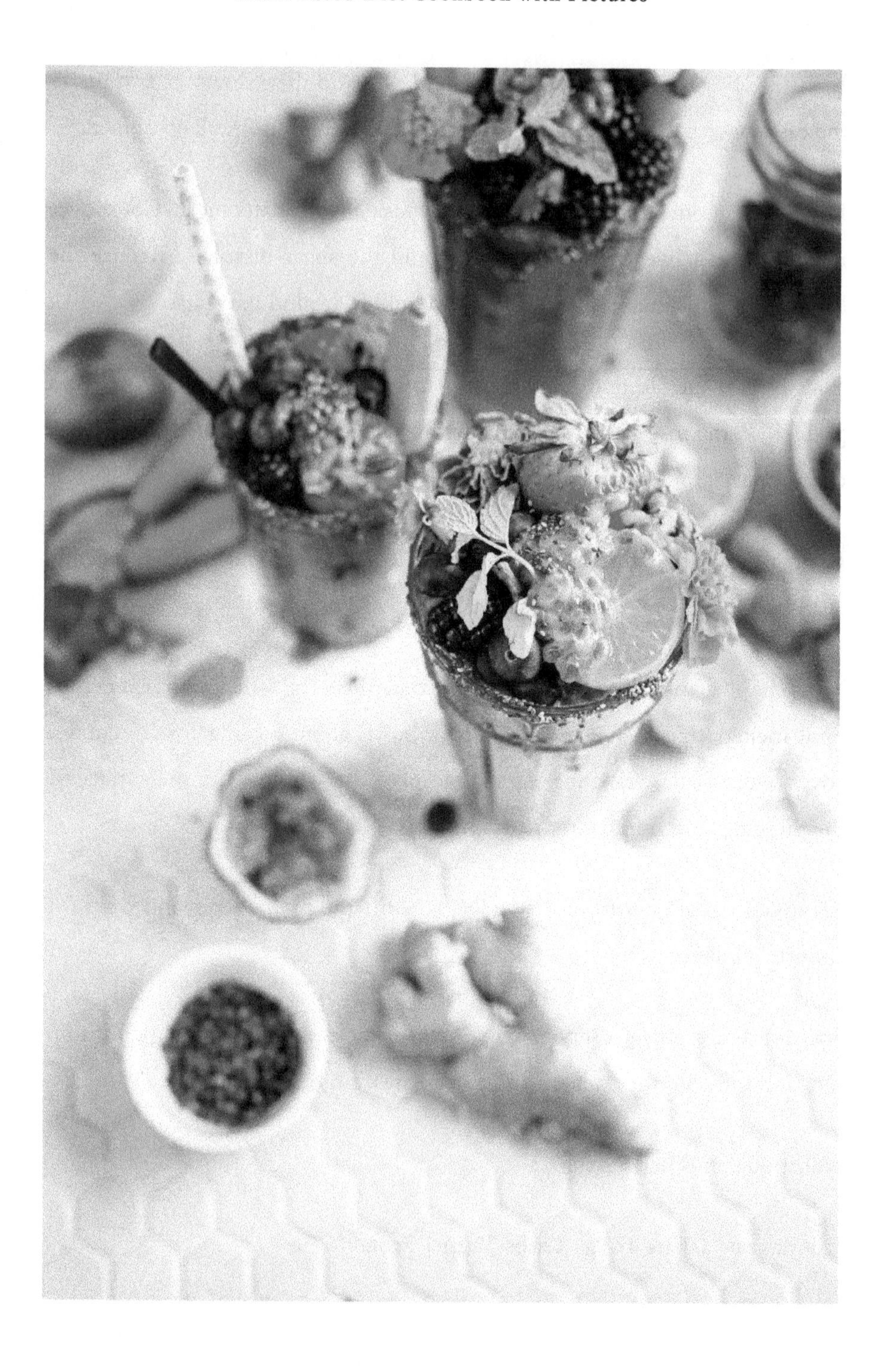

Quick Energy & Recovery Snacks

43. Spiced Chickpeas

Preparation Time: 45 Minutes Cooking Time: 40 minutes

Servings: 4

Ingredients:

Cayenne Pepper (.10 t.)

Dried Oregano (.25 t.)

Garlic Powder (.10 t.)

Salt (to Taste)

Olive Oil (2 T.)

Chickpeas (1 Can)

Directions:

Start this recipe by prepping the oven to 450 and lining a baking sheet with parchment paper. Take a mixing bowl, add in chickpeas and coat with the spices and olive oil. Once this is done, pop everything into the oven for 40 minutes. After 40 minutes, remove the pan from the oven, allow it to cool completely and enjoy.

Nutrition: Calories: 170 Proteins: 7g Carbs: 31g Fats: 2g

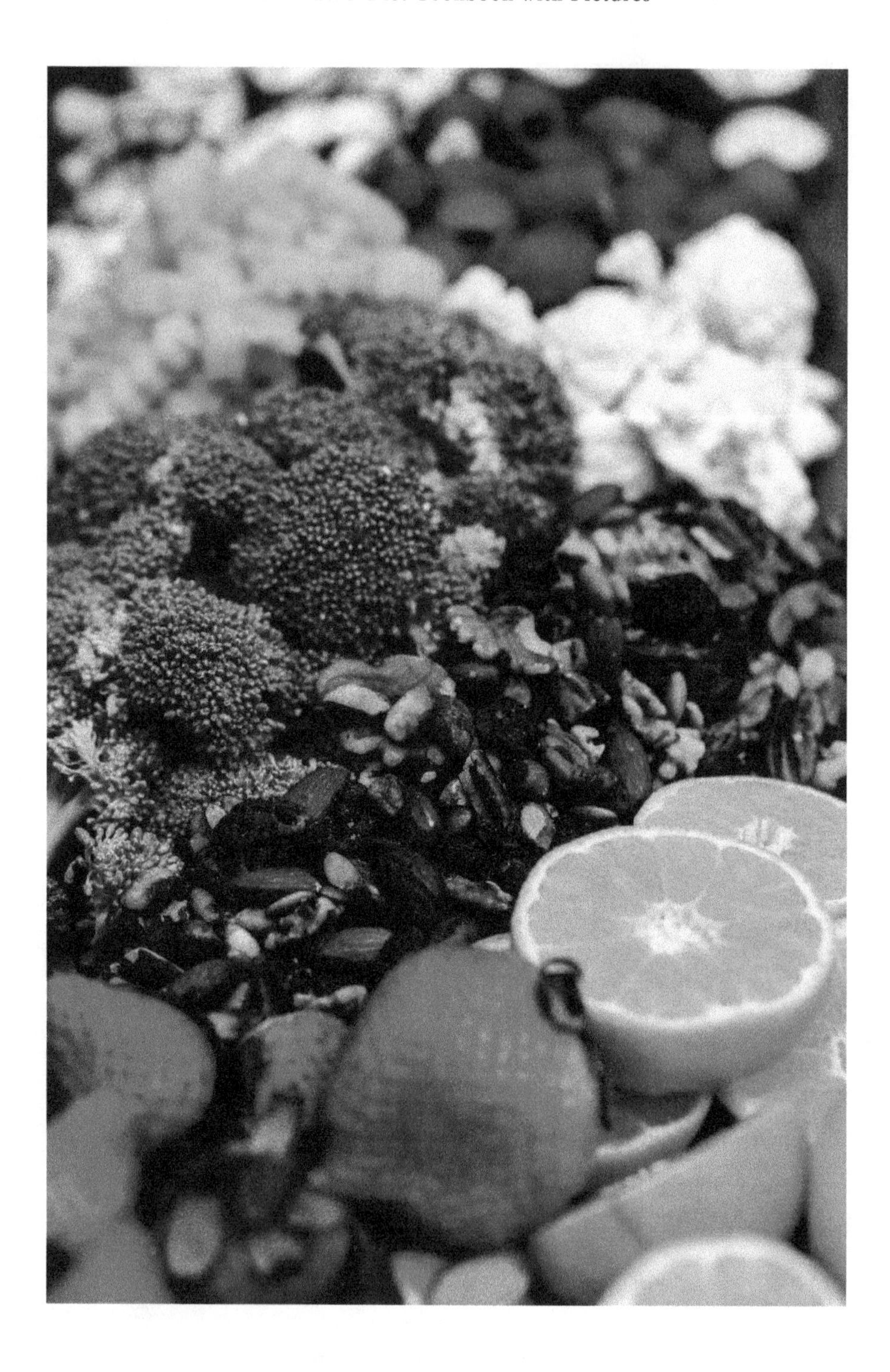

Flavour Boosters (Fish Glazes, Meat Rubs & Fish Rubs)

44. Classic Honey Mustard Fish Glaze

Complement your choice of fish including salmon by infusing it with succulent flavors and a perfectly glazed look by this classic honey mustard glaze.

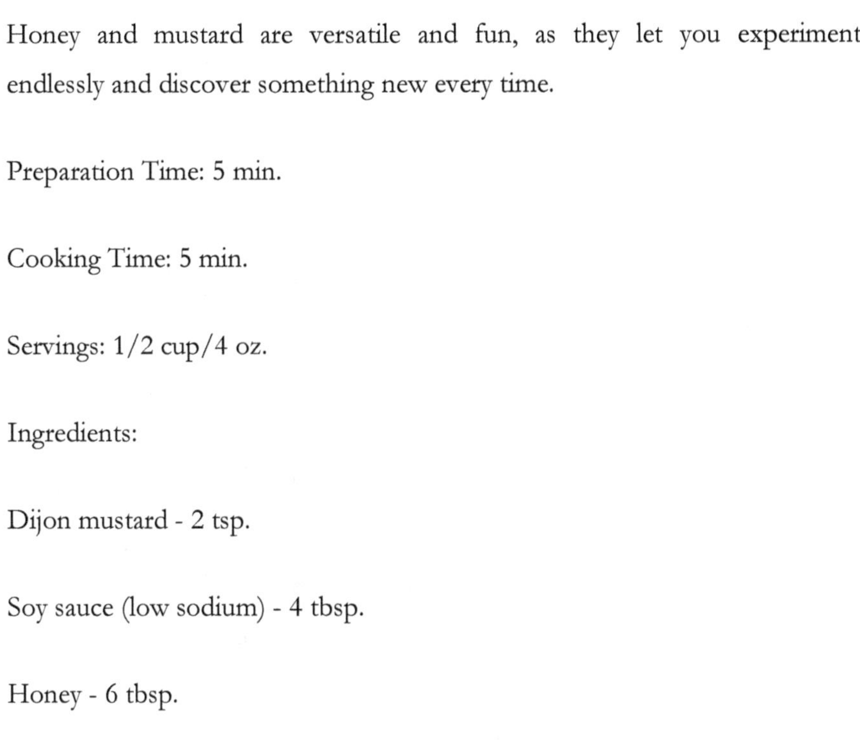

Honey and mustard are versatile and fun, as they let you experiment endlessly and discover something new every time.

Preparation Time: 5 min.

Cooking Time: 5 min.

Servings: 1/2 cup/4 oz.

Ingredients:

Dijon mustard - 2 tsp.

Soy sauce (low sodium) - 4 tbsp.

Honey - 6 tbsp.

Lime juice - 2 tsp.

Directions:

To make the honey mustard fish glaze, combine the mustard, soy sauce, lime juice, and honey in your medium-sized bowl. Gently blend the ingredients.

Then, add the mixture into your medium-sized saucepan. Let the mixture simmer gradually for about 2 minutes.

Now, take your favorite cooked/grilled/baked salmon or any other fish variety. Gently spread or pour the prepared glaze over the fish/salmon. Allow a few minutes for the glaze to set in. Enjoy the mustard glazed fish meal!

45. Maple Syrup Spiced Fish Glaze

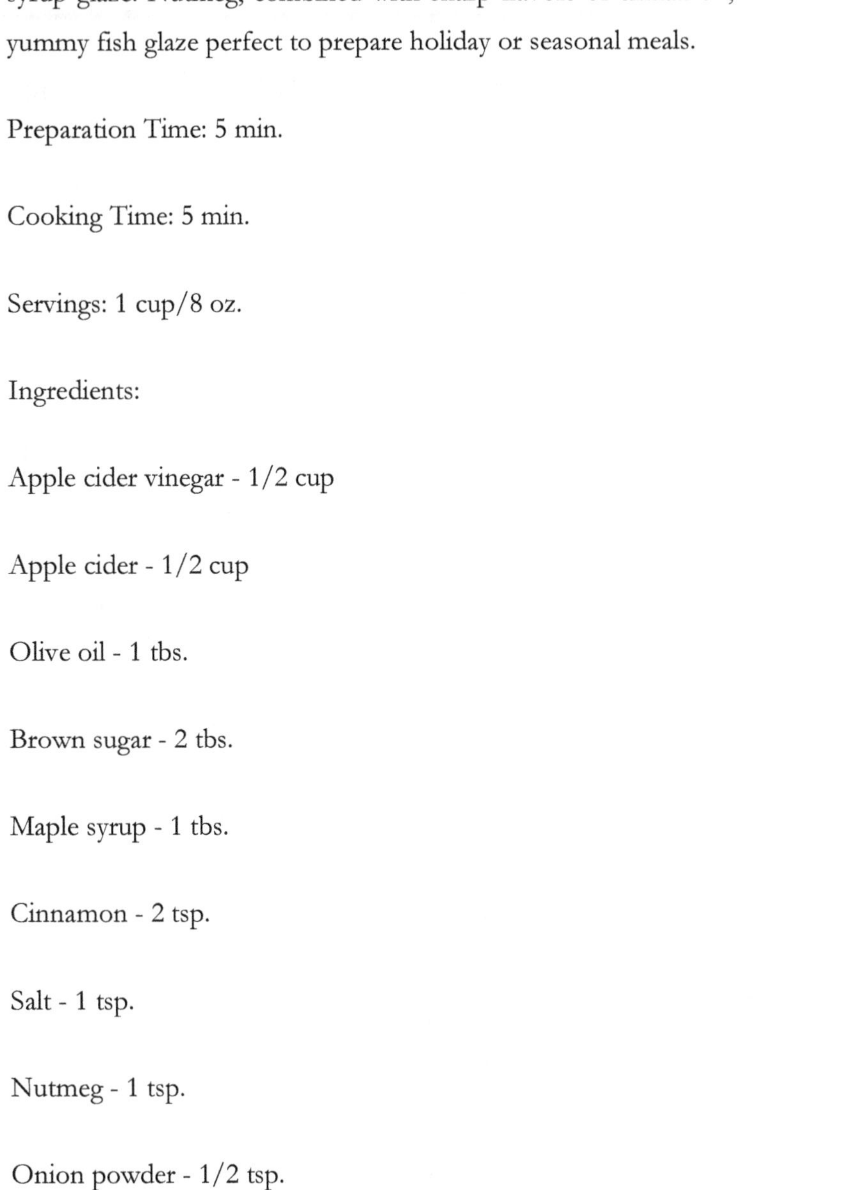

Give your parties and occasions a rich and classic upgrade with this maple syrup glaze. Nutmeg, combined with sharp flavors of cinnamon, makes this yummy fish glaze perfect to prepare holiday or seasonal meals.

Preparation Time: 5 min.

Cooking Time: 5 min.

Servings: 1 cup/8 oz.

Ingredients:

Apple cider vinegar - 1/2 cup

Apple cider - 1/2 cup

Olive oil - 1 tbs.

Brown sugar - 2 tbs.

Maple syrup - 1 tbs.

Cinnamon - 2 tsp.

Salt - 1 tsp.

Nutmeg - 1 tsp.

Onion powder - 1/2 tsp.

Directions:

To make the maple syrup glaze, combine all mentioned fish marinade ingredients in your food processor or blender. Gently blend the ingredients.

Now, take your favorite cooked/grilled/baked baked salmon or any other fish variety. Gently spread or pour the prepared glaze over the cuts. Allow a few minutes for the glaze to set in. Enjoy the maple syrup-glazed fish meal!

46. Lemon Pepper Coriander Rub

This intelligently created pepper coriander rub provides hints of tartness along with mild spiciness with inclusion of chili powder. A great choice of rub to flavor-up your weekend nights as well as any night you wish to make special.

Partner your fish meals prepared with this special rub with red wine for a truly refreshing meal time.

Preparation Time: 5 min.

Cooking Time: 5 min.

Servings: ½ cup + 3 tsp.

Ingredients:

Chili powder - 1 tbsp.

Lemon pepper seasoning - 1/4 cup

Ground cumin - 1 tbsp.

Light brown sugar, firmly packed - 1 1/2 tsp.

Ground coriander - 1 tbsp.

Kosher salt - 1/2 tsp.

Ground black pepper - 1 1/4 tsp.

Red pepper flakes - 1/2 tsp.

Directions:

Mix in all mentioned ingredients in your mixing bowl to make the lemon coriander rub. Gently mix all the ingredients using spatula or spoon to form an aromatic rub mixture.

Now, take your choice of fish and place it on a firm surface. Brush or rub the freshly made rub on it; pat gently for the rub onto stick on the surface. Turn it and repeat to spice up its other side.

Let your fish cuts adequately season for more rich flavors for some time in your refrigerator.

*Do not let your fish season for more than 2 hours (but not less than 30 minutes).

Take it out, as it is ready to be cooked or grilled!

Sauce Recipes

47. Runner Recovery Bites

Preparation time: 10 minutes

Cooking time: 10 minutes

Servings: 12

Ingredients:

1/4 cup pumpkin seeds, soaked for 1 hour

1/3 cup oats

1/4 cup sunflower seeds, soaked for 1 hour

5 dates

1 teaspoon maca powder

1 tablespoon goji berries

1 teaspoon coconut, shredded and unsweetened

1 tablespoon coconut water

1 teaspoon vanilla extract

1 tablespoon protein powder

1 tablespoon maple syrup

1/4 cup hemp seeds

A pinch sea salt

Directions:

Drain sunflower and pumpkin seeds and add to a blender. Blend until a paste forms. Add dates and blend to mix. Add the remaining ingredients except hemp seeds and blend until a dough forms.

Roll 1 tablespoon dough into balls with hands. Roll the ball in hemp seeds until covered.

Transfer the prepared balls to a plate and freeze until firm.

Serve and enjoy.

Meal Plans

48. Meal Plan 1

Day	Breakfast	Lunch	Dinner	Snacks
1	Chocolate PB Smoothie	Cauliflower Latke	Noodles Alfredo with Herby Tofu	Beans with Sesame Hummus
2	Orange french toast	Roasted Brussels Sprouts	Lemon Couscous with Tempeh Kabobs	Candied Honey-Coconut Peanuts
3	Oatmeal Raisin Breakfast Cookie	Brussels Sprouts & Cranberries Salad	Portobello Burger with Veggie Fries	Choco Walnuts Fat Bombs
4	Berry Beetsicle Smoothie	Potato Latke	Thai Seitan Vegetable Curry	Crispy Honey Pecans (Slow Cooker)
5	Blueberry Oat Muffins	Broccoli Rabe	Tofu Cabbage Stir-Fry	Crunchy Fried Pickles
6	Quinoa Applesauce Muffins	Whipped Potatoes	Curried Tofu with Buttery Cabbage	Granola bars with Maple Syrup
7	Pumpkin	Quinoa	Smoked Tempeh with	Green Soy

	pancakes	Avocado Salad	Broccoli Fritters	Beans Hummus
8	Green breakfast smoothie	Roasted Sweet Potatoes	Cheesy Potato Casserole	High Protein Avocado Guacamole
9	Blueberry Lemonade Smoothie	Cauliflower Salad	Curry Mushroom Pie	Homemade Energy Nut Bars
10	Berry Protein Smoothie	Garlic Mashed Potatoes & Turnips	Spicy Cheesy Tofu Balls	Honey Peanut Butter
11	Blueberry and chia smoothie	Green Beans with Bacon	Radish Chips	Mediterranean Marinated Olives
12	Green Kickstart Smoothie	Coconut Brussels Sprouts	Sautéed Pears	Nut Butter & Dates Granola
13	Warm Maple and Cinnamon Quinoa	Cod Stew with Rice & Sweet Potatoes	Pecan & Blueberry Crumble	Oven-baked Caramelize Plantains
14	Warm Quinoa Breakfast Bowl	Chicken & Rice	Rice Pudding	Powerful Peas & Lentils Dip
15	Banana Bread	Rice Bowl with	Mango Sticky	Protein "Raffaello"

	Rice Pudding	Edamame	Rice	Candies
16	Apple and cinnamon oatmeal	Chickpea Avocado Sandwich	Noodles Alfredo with Herby Tofu	Protein-Rich Pumpkin Bowl
17	Mango Key Lime Pie Smoothie	Roasted Tomato Sandwich	Lemon Couscous with Tempeh Kabobs	Savory Red Potato-Garlic Balls
18	Spiced orange breakfast couscous	Pulled "Pork" Sandwiches	Portobello Burger with Veggie Fries	Spicy Smooth Red Lentil Dip
19	Breakfast parfaits	Cauliflower Latke	Thai Seitan Vegetable Curry	Steamed Broccoli with Sesame
20	Sweet potato and kale hash	Roasted Brussels Sprouts	Tofu Cabbage Stir-Fry	Vegan Eggplant Patties
21	Delicious Oat Meal	Brussels Sprouts & Cranberries Salad	Curried Tofu with Buttery Cabbage	Vegan Breakfast Sandwich
22	Breakfast Cherry Delight	Potato Latke	Smoked Tempeh with Broccoli	Chickpea And Mushroom Burger

			Fritters	
23	Crazy Maple and Pear Breakfast	Broccoli Rabe	Cheesy Potato Casserole	Beans with Sesame Hummus
24	Hearty French Toast Bowls	Whipped Potatoes	Curry Mushroom Pie	Candied Honey-Coconut Peanuts
25	Chocolate PB Smoothie	Quinoa Avocado Salad	Spicy Cheesy Tofu Balls	Choco Walnuts Fat Bombs
26	Orange french toast	Roasted Sweet Potatoes	Radish Chips	Crispy Honey Pecans (Slow Cooker)
27	Oatmeal Raisin Breakfast Cookie	Cauliflower Salad	Sautéed Pears	Crunchy Fried Pickles
28	Berry Beetsicle Smoothie	Garlic Mashed Potatoes & Turnips	Pecan & Blueberry Crumble	Granola bars with Maple Syrup

49. Meal Plan 2

Day	Breakfast	Lunch	Dinner	Smoothie
1	Mexican-Spiced Tofu Scramble	Teriyaki Tofu Stir-fry	Mushroom Steak	Chocolate Smoothie
2	Whole Grain Protein Bowl	Red Lentil and Quinoa Fritters	Spicy Grilled Tofu Steak	Chocolate Mint Smoothie
3	Healthy Breakfast Bowl	Green Pea Fritters	Piquillo Salsa Verde Steak	Cinnamon Roll Smoothie
4	Healthy Breakfast Bowl	Breaded Tofu Steaks	Butternut Squash Steak	Coconut Smoothie
5	Root Vegetable Hash With Avocado Crème	Chickpea and Edamame Salad	Cauliflower Steak Kicking Corn	Maca Almond Smoothie
6	Chocolate Strawberry Almond Protein Smoothie	Thai Tofu and Quinoa Bowls	Pistachio Watermelon Steak	Blueberry Smoothie
7	Banana Bread Breakfast Muffins	Black Bean and Bulgur Chili	BBQ Ribs	Nutty Protein Shake
8	Stracciatella Muffins	Cauliflower Steaks	Spicy Veggie Steaks With veggies	Cinnamon Pear Smoothie
9	Cardamom Persimmon Scones With	Avocado and Hummus	Mushroom Steak	Vanilla Milkshake

	Maple-Persimmon Cream	Sandwich		
10	Activated Buckwheat & Coconut Porridge With Blueberry Sauce	Chickpea Spinach Salad	Spicy Grilled Tofu Steak	Raspberry Protein Shake
11	Sweet Molasses Brown Bread	Teriyaki Tofu Stir-fry	Piquillo Salsa Verde Steak	Raspberry Almond Smoothie
12	Mexican-Spiced Tofu Scramble	Red Lentil and Quinoa Fritters	Butternut Squash Steak	Chocolate Smoothie
13	Whole Grain Protein Bowl	Green Pea Fritters	Cauliflower Steak Kicking Corn	Chocolate Mint Smoothie
14	Healthy Breakfast Bowl	Breaded Tofu Steaks	Pistachio Watermelon Steak	Cinnamon Roll Smoothie
15	Healthy Breakfast Bowl	Chickpea and Edamame Salad	BBQ Ribs	Coconut Smoothie
16	Root Vegetable Hash With Avocado Crème	Thai Tofu and Quinoa Bowls	Spicy Veggie Steaks With veggies	Maca Almond Smoothie
17	Chocolate Strawberry Almond Protein	Black Bean and Bulgur Chili	Mushroom Steak	Blueberry Smoothie

	Smoothie			
18	Banana Bread Breakfast Muffins	Cauliflower Steaks	Spicy Grilled Tofu Steak	Nutty Protein Shake
19	Stracciatella Muffins	Avocado and Hummus Sandwich	Piquillo Salsa Verde Steak	Cinnamon Pear Smoothie
20	Cardamom Persimmon Scones With Maple-Persimmon Cream	Chickpea Spinach Salad	Butternut Squash Steak	Vanilla Milkshake
21	Activated Buckwheat & Coconut Porridge With Blueberry Sauce	Teriyaki Tofu Stir-fry	Cauliflower Steak Kicking Corn	Raspberry Protein Shake
22	Sweet Molasses Brown Bread	Red Lentil and Quinoa Fritters	Pistachio Watermelon Steak	Raspberry Almond Smoothie
23	Mexican-Spiced Tofu Scramble	Green Pea Fritters	BBQ Ribs	Chocolate Smoothie
24	Whole Grain Protein Bowl	Breaded Tofu Steaks	Spicy Veggie Steaks With veggies	Chocolate Mint Smoothie

25	Healthy Breakfast Bowl	Chickpea and Edamame Salad	Mushroom Steak	Cinnamon Roll Smoothie
26	Healthy Breakfast Bowl	Thai Tofu and Quinoa Bowls	Spicy Grilled Tofu Steak	Coconut Smoothie
27	Root Vegetable Hash With Avocado Crème	Black Bean and Bulgur Chili	Piquillo Salsa Verde Steak	Maca Almond Smoothie
28	Chocolate Strawberry Almond Protein Smoothie	Cauliflower Steaks	Butternut Squash Steak	Blueberry Smoothie

50. Meal Plan 3

Day	Breakfast	Lunch	Dinner	Snacks
1	Breakfast Blueberry Muffins	Quinoa Buddha Bowl	Broccoli & black beans stir fry	Spiced Chickpeas
2	Oatmeal with Pears	Lettuce Hummus Wrap	Stuffed peppers	Lemon & Ginger Kale Chips
3	Yogurt with Cucumber	Simple Curried Vegetable Rice	Sweet 'n spicy tofu	Chocolate Energy Snack Bar
4	Breakfast Casserole	Spicy Southwestern Hummus Wraps	Eggplant & mushrooms in peanut sauce	Hazelnut & Maple Chia Crunch
5	Berries with Mascarpone on Toasted Bread	Buffalo Cauliflower Wings	Green beans stir fry	Roasted Cauliflower
6	Fruit Cup	Veggie Fritters	Collard greens 'n tofu	Apple Cinnamon Crisps
7	Oatmeal with Black Beans & Cheddar	Pizza Bites	Cassoulet	Pumpkin Spice Granola Bites
8	Breakfast Smoothie	Avocado, Spinach and Kale Soup	Double-garlic bean and vegetable soup	Salted Carrot Fries
9	Yogurt with Beets & Raspberries	Curry spinach soup	Mean bean minestrone	Zesty Orange Muffins

10	Curry Oatmeal	Arugula and Artichokes Bowls	Grilled Halloumi Broccoli Salad	Chocolate Tahini Balls
11	Fig & Cheese Oatmeal	Minty arugula soup	Black Bean Lentil Salad With Lime Dressing	Spiced Chickpeas
12	Pumpkin Oats	Spinach and Broccoli Soup	Arugula Lentil Salad	Lemon & Ginger Kale Chips
13	Sweet Potato Toasts	Coconut zucchini cream	Red Cabbage Salad With Curried Seitan	Chocolate Energy Snack Bar
14	Tofu Scramble Tacos	Zucchini and Cauliflower Soup	Chickpea, Red Kidney Bean And Feta Salad	Hazelnut & Maple Chia Crunch
15	Almond Chia Pudding	Chard soup	The Amazing Chickpea Spinach Salad	Roasted Cauliflower
16	Breakfast Parfait Popsicles	Avocado, Pine Nuts and Chard Salad	Curried Carrot Slaw With Tempeh	Apple Cinnamon Crisps
17	Strawberry Smoothie Bowl	Grapes, Avocado and Spinach Salad	Black & White Bean Quinoa Salad	Pumpkin Spice Granola Bites
18	Peanut Butter Granola	Greens and Olives Pan	Greek Salad With Seitan Gyros Strips	Salted Carrot Fries
19	Apple Chia Pudding	Mushrooms and Chard Soup	Chickpea And Edamame Salad	Zesty Orange Muffins
20	Pumpkin Spice Bites	Tomato, Green Beans and Chard	Broccoli & black beans stir fry	Chocolate Tahini Balls

		Soup		
21	Lemon Spelt Scones	Hot roasted peppers cream	Stuffed peppers	Spiced Chickpeas
22	Veggie Breakfast Scramble	Eggplant and Peppers Soup	Sweet 'n spicy tofu	Lemon & Ginger Kale Chips
23	Breakfast Blueberry Muffins	Eggplant and Olives Stew	Eggplant & mushrooms in peanut sauce	Chocolate Energy Snack Bar
24	Oatmeal with Pears	Cauliflower and Artichokes Soup	Green beans stir fry	Hazelnut & Maple Chia Crunch
25	Yogurt with Cucumber	Quinoa Buddha Bowl	Collard greens 'n tofu	Roasted Cauliflower
26	Breakfast Casserole	Lettuce Hummus Wrap	Cassoulet	Apple Cinnamon Crisps
27	Berries with Mascarpone on Toasted Bread	Simple Curried Vegetable Rice	Double-garlic bean and vegetable soup	Pumpkin Spice Granola Bites
28	Fruit Cup	Spicy Southwestern Hummus Wraps	Mean bean minestrone	Salted Carrot Fries

51. Meal plan 4

Day	Breakfast	Entrées	Soup , Salad, & Sides	Smoothie
1	Tasty Oatmeal Muffins	Black Bean Dip	Spinach Soup with Dill and Basil	Fruity Smoothie
2	Omelet with Chickpea Flour	Cannellini Bean Cashew Dip	Coconut Watercress Soup	Energizing Ginger Detox Tonic
3	White Sandwich Bread	Cauliflower Popcorn	Coconut Watercress Soup	Warm Spiced Lemon Drink
4	A Toast to Remember	Cinnamon Apple Chips with Dip	Coconut Watercress Soup	Soothing Ginger Tea Drink
5	Tasty Panini	Crunchy Asparagus Spears	Cauliflower Spinach Soup	Nice Spiced Cherry Cider
6	Tasty Oatmeal and Carrot Cake	Cucumber Bites with Chive and Sunflower Seeds	Avocado Mint Soup	Fragrant Spiced Coffee

7	Onion & Mushroom Tart with a Nice Brown Rice Crust	Garlicky Kale Chips	Creamy Squash Soup	Tangy Spiced Cranberry Drink
8	Perfect Breakfast Shake	Hummus-stuffed Baby Potatoes	Cucumber Edamame Salad	Warm Pomegranate Punch
9	Beet Gazpacho	Homemade Trail Mix	Best Broccoli Salad	Rich Truffle Hot Chocolate
10	Vegetable Rice	Nut Butter Maple Dip	Rainbow Orzo Salad	Ultimate Mulled Wine
11	Courgette Risotto	Oven Baked Sesame Fries	Broccoli Pasta Salad	Pleasant Lemonade
12	Country Breakfast Cereal	Pumpkin Orange Spice Hummus	Eggplant & Roasted Tomato Farro Salad	Pineapple, Banana & Spinach Smoothie
13	Oatmeal Fruit Shake	Quick English Muffin Mexican Pizzas	Garden Patch Sandwiches on Multigrain Bread	Kale & Avocado Smoothie
14	Amaranth Banana Breakfast	Quinoa Trail Mix Cups	Garden Salad Wraps	Coconut & Strawberry Smoothie

	Porridge			
15	Green Ginger Smoothie	Black Bean Dip	Marinated Mushroom Wraps	Pumpkin Chia Smoothie
16	Orange Dream Creamsicle	Cannellini Bean Cashew Dip	Tamari Toasted Almonds	Cantaloupe Smoothie Bowl
17	Strawberry Limeade	Cauliflower Popcorn	Nourishing Whole-Grain Porridge	Berry & Cauliflower Smoothie
18	Peanut Butter and Jelly Smoothie	Cinnamon Apple Chips with Dip	Pungent Mushroom Barley Risotto	Green Mango Smoothie
19	Banana Almond Granola	Crunchy Asparagus Spears	Spinach Soup with Dill and Basil	Chia Seed Smoothie
20	Tasty Oatmeal Muffins	Cucumber Bites with Chive and Sunflower Seeds	Coconut Watercress Soup	Mango Smoothie
21	Omelet with Chickpea Flour	Garlicky Kale Chips	Coconut Watercress Soup	Fruity Smoothie

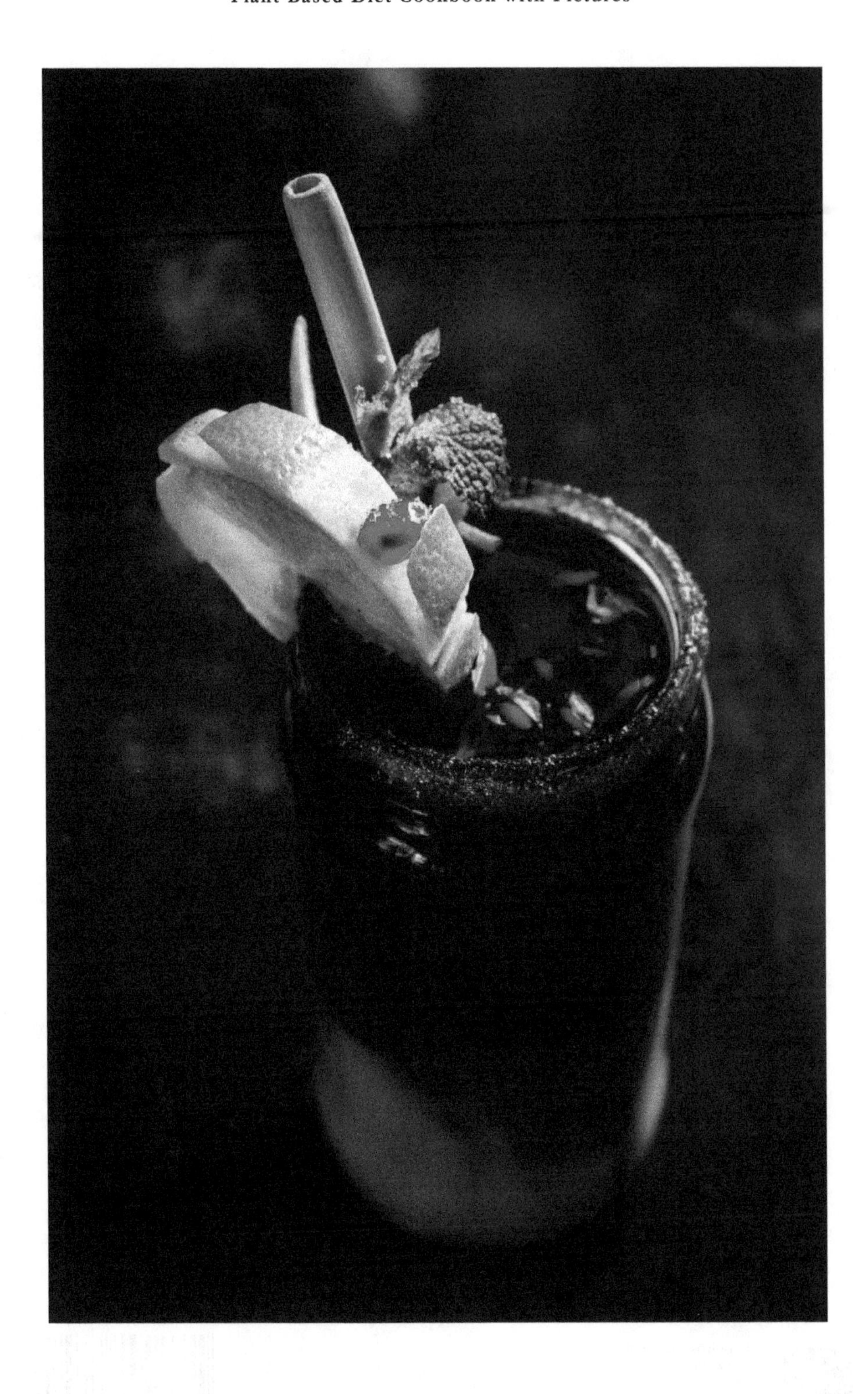

CPSIA information can be obtained
at www.ICGtesting.com
Printed in the USA
BVHW062006250321
603411BV00002B/95